Love Never Fails

Praise for Four Women & The Appeal of Ebony Jones

"The characters may be fictional, but the problems are real and relevant in this period of #SurvivingRKelly and #BlackLivesMatter. The issues the women in this book face are not exclusive to Black communities but it does challenge the notion of people not taking the pain experienced by Black women to be serious."

— REWRITE London

"It's a sobering and chilling story . . . this book will make you see the world through the eyes of at least one of these black women — and it's a different world, indeed."

— *Creative Loafing Tampa*

"Williams . . . places her readers inside the very complex contemporary lives her characters lead: from reformed-ish parents to the intricacies of female friendships in the workplace. In this, it's also a deeply human commentary on race, policing and justice in America."

— *Folio Weekly*

"Williams exhibits her ambitious nature by the subject matter she chose to tackle in her debut novel, which includes domestic violence, sexual abuse, bigotry, and the abuse of power."

— Cultural Council of Greater Jacksonville

"[The Appeal of Ebony Jones] examines how the justice system treats women who are themselves victims, specifically women of color. It also examines female friendships, and how adversity can play a role in those relationships."
—*Void Magazine*

"The dilemma in [Four Women] is the question can justice be served when the suspect is also the victim?"
— P.R.I.D.E Book Club

Also By Nikesha Elise Williams

Four Women
The Appeal of Ebony Jones

TED Talks

Pregnancy is Inconvenient — TEDxFSU (March 2018)
Representation Matters — TEDxFSCJ (April 2018)

Love Never Fails

Nikesha Elise Williams

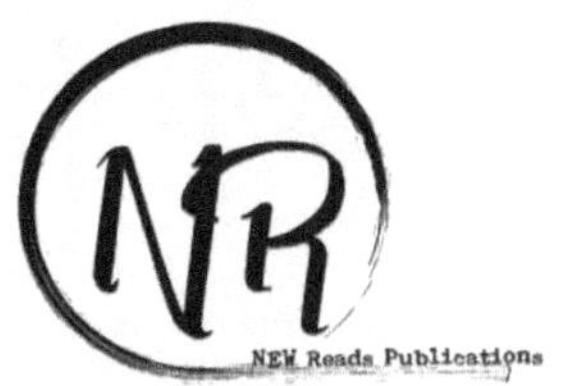

Library of Congress Cataloging-In-Publication Data

Williams, Nikesha Elise.
    Love Never Fails/Nikesha Elise Williams

    ISBN 978-1-7335848-0-7

PUBLISHER'S NOTE
This book is a work of fiction. Names, characters, places, and incidents and circumstances are the product of the author's imagination or are used fictitiously. Any resemblance to actual persons, living or dead, business establishments, events, or locales is entirely coincidental.

For Jermaine

Love is patient, love is kind. It does not envy, it does not boast, it is not proud. It does not dishonor others, it is not self-seeking, it is not easily angered, it keeps no record of wrongs. Love does not delight in evil but rejoices with the truth. It always protects, always trusts, always hopes, always perseveres.

Love never fails.

1 Corinthians 13:4-8

1.

If I were honest, I'd be divorced right now.

The words jump off the page in front of Jolene's eyes. Her truth is startling, even to herself. She puts the inky pen back to the paper of her gold lined journal and writes.

It's not that what we have is bad, it's just the same. The same old routine. The same old jobs, the same old sex, the same old arguments. The same old "I'm sorry's" after so we don't go to bed mad. It's the same. If I had known monogamy was synonymous with monotony, I would have never signed up for this. Never said "I do." But who am I kidding? I was thirsty to get married. Being a single parent was hard enough; might as well let somebody else carry this burden with me. And I guess that's the thing that keeps me here. Still in Jacksonville. Damn near in the same neighborhood I grew up in, with the only other person that's ever really cared about me besides my family. I just don't know how long I can keep hoping, wishing, waiting, praying, for that spark to come back between us. But, Mo has always been good with Toussaint. Always treated him like his own son, even when Jemarcus was in the picture.

Even right now, I can hear them downstairs. I'm supposed to be in the tub, but sometimes I just need to sit down and gather my thoughts without doing anything else. Including bathing. I'll wash eventually. But just sitting here, listening to them downstairs, Mo helping Toussaint with his homework, with Lydia yelling "Daddy, Daddy, Daddy" every five minutes, he's determined to get that boy through Algebra. That's better than I can do. I barely passed that class myself. All those y's and x's and numbers together, might as well be Wookiee. I don't understand it. I didn't when I was in school and I still don't. I teach history. It never changes. We just have to learn from it.

"TeeTee, you got it?"

Jolene hears Mosiah ask Toussaint as he comes up the stairs to their bedroom.

"Yeah, I got it," Toussaint answers.

"Then I'm a take a shower. Keep an eye on your sister."

Jolene braces herself against the bed pillows. Her head is laid back against the upholstered headboard the color of red wine. She drops her pen in the journal and closes the soft leather book. *I'll finish this later,* she promises herself. She closes her eyes as Mosiah comes into the room. She can feel him looking at her in the doorway.

"I thought you were getting in the tub," he says.

"I am. I just needed to unwind first."

"You know the kids are hungry? Elmo's only going to hold Lydia for so long."

"I know. I'm coming. I just needed a minute."

"You've been up here for an hour."

"Okay, I needed an hour," Jolene snaps. "I'll take a shower and go cook."

"You know we can just order in," Mosiah suggests.

"Yeah, I know, but I just went grocery shopping. It's cheaper to feed the four of us from what I gave the store than anything we have delivered from Uber Eats."

"I was just trying to help you out," Mosiah says, coming toward the bed.

"You did. You helped Toussaint with his math homework. For that I'm forever grateful."

"You're welcome."

Mosiah holds out his hands to Jolene. She swings her feet off the bed, takes his hands and stands up. She stumbles into his arms.

"Woah," he says, wrapping his arms around her back. "You alright?"

"Yeah. I just got dizzy on the way up."

"Lay your head down, I'll hold you as long as you need me to."

Jolene nestles her head into his neck. She inhales his scent. The smell of industrial disinfectant and Clinique aftershave clouds her senses. She turns her head away from his body and sees the abstract artworks they bought from a Home Goods store to add a level of maturity to their bedroom. She stares at the tan canvases with splashes and splotches of vibrant paint until the reds bleed into the yellows, the browns into the greens, and the purples into the blues. Her gaze lingers until her level of dizziness increases and she stumbles even more into Mosiah, nearly knocking him over.

He catches his step and holds on to her even tighter.

He says, "Baby, what's wrong?"

"I'm just tired." Jolene fakes a yawn. "But I'm alright. Let me jump in the shower and clear my head, then I can get dinner together."

"I can do it," Mosiah offers.

"You've had a long day too. We both have. I got it."

Jolene steps out of Mosiah's arms and walks into their small closet. She begins to take off her clothes. She pulls the purple split-neck blouse over her head, messing up her long, straight hair along the way. She smooths the sides back around her face before spinning her black pencil skirt around her waist to take it off. First the button, then the zipper, and she still has to pull it inch by inch away from her hips and down her thighs, until it falls from her knees to the floor. Jolene runs her fingers through the silver hooks of her waist trainer until it falls away from her body. She puts her hands on her hips and exhales deeply.

"I don't know why you insist on wearing all that everyday," Mosiah says.

"You know it's rude to stand in the doorway just staring at people like a creeper," Jolene says without turning around.

"Not if I'm staring at my wife."

"Whatever." She blows out more air.

"That's probably why you're dizzy," he says, coming to stand beside her. "Barely breathing all day has probably got you light headed. The body needs to breathe."

"Are you some sort of doctor now?"

"You don't have to be a doctor to know that without breath we die."

He unzips his navy blue janitorial suit, pulls the sleeves off of his arms, and steps out of it. Jolene notices the patch with his company logo is coming off one of the sides. Mosiah picks up the dirty suit from the carpeted floor and balls it up to toss it into the dark brown, wicker dirty clothes hamper.

"Don't," she says, holding out her hand. "Your patch is loose. Let me take it to the cleaners and have them put it back on. They can clean it, too, so it'll be fresh the next time you wear it."

"Okay. I have two more hanging up. I'll press one tonight for tomorrow."

Jolene takes the suit from his hands, careful to not disturb the loose patch on the front left corner. She rubs her thumb over the thickly threaded cursive lettering that reads "The Walker Way Cleaning Service." The company Mosiah started after Lydia was born, when he decided cutting heads as a barber wasn't enough to keep the bills paid, and have enough discretionary spending money on the side.

"Jo, I gotta do something else," she remembers him saying to her.

With Lydia nursing at her breast, she asked him, "Why? You make good money at the shop. And I do alright at the school. We have everything we need. Why do you want to clean buildings?"

He said to her, "I want more than just what we need. I want to have whatever I want, you, whatever you want, whatever TeeTee or this little one here wants."

She said, "Okay then. Go ahead. You have my support."

"Then, I know it's going to be a success," he said, kissing her nose and then her lips and then baby Lydia's forehead.

Jolene smiles at the memory, still holding the jumpsuit caressing the logo.

"You coming," Mosiah says, peeking his head into the closet.

"You're in the shower already? I didn't even see you walk out. Let me get the rest of this off."

She throws the balled up jumpsuit beside the hamper with a few of her dresses that need to be dry cleaned, and starts to work on her Spanx.

"Let me help you with that," Mosiah says, walking up behind her.

"Boy, you're naked."

"As the day I was born," he says, pulling down the thin straps of her black body suit.

Mosiah pulls the suit all the way down to Jolene's feet until he is on one knee, and the suit is inside out as she steps out of it. He runs his rough hands up her legs, over her dimpled thighs, and across her butt, admiring the stretch mark stripes he calls her lines of wisdom, cut through her caramel colored skin. The lines and dimples from her hips to her waist that show she has left behind adolescence, and the wiles of a young woman, and is fully grown with the weight and scars to prove it.

He places a gentle kiss on the fattest part of her behind.

"What are you doing back there?" She looks down at him over her shoulder.

"I'm helping, I told you."

Mosiah pulls the frilly fabric of her purple panties that barely hold all of her in down, over her hips, ass, and legs until they fall to the floor with the shape wear and her skirt. Jolene reaches behind her back to unclasp her bra.

"I didn't ask you to do that," Mosiah says.

She drops her hands to her sides.

He stands behind her and unhooks the matching purple demi-cup bra. Pulling it off her back and away from her shoulders, he drops it to the floor. His hands sink into the softness of her flesh around her waist and he spins her around to face him.

"What are you doing?" Jolene asks.

He puts one of his long index fingers to her lips and says, "I want to tell you, how beautiful you are."

Jolene heaves a heavy sigh. *It's always the same. Here we go.*

"Thank you," she says, dipping her head in embarrassed annoyance.

Mosiah lifts her chin and kisses her lips. He eases into the kiss taking his time, paying close attention to the pillowy softness of her lips and the warmth of her tongue. He kisses her and pulls her body in closer to his, wrapping his arms tighter around her waist, his hands on her ass, gripping the weight of her bountiful gift.

Breaking the kiss at her mouth, he kisses his way down her body. His wet lips brush past her chin, collar bone, and between her breasts and navel to the top of her yoni. His hands grip the underside of her ass as he pulls her closer still, burying his face in her womb. Mosiah kisses and licks her outer and inner lips until his work is repaid with the sweetness of her honey, moistening the top of his mouth.

Jolene looks down on his head. His eyes are closed, intent on delivering pleasure. She cups the back of his head and holds it to one spot to allow the persistent pressure to build in her body that will force her to let go of the days stress. A subtle moan escapes her lips as she relinquishes her anxiety and her discomfort with being too comfortable. *Give in*, she demands of herself. *He's a good man*, she tells herself. *Any other woman would happily trade places with you and fuck him six ways from Sunday, if she had to.*

Jolene lifts one leg from the floor and places it on his thigh, giving Mosiah more access to all of her. Without moving his mouth, he reaches both arms under her butt and lifts her off the floor as he stands to his feet. He sucks and licks at her fleshy folds as he walks her to their bed. Jolene holds his head, closes her eyes, and gives in to the woman inside craving for release.

Mosiah lowers Jolene to the bedspread and continues his quest in cunnilingus to make his wife speak in soft tongues and rude words she never wants him to hear her say.

He doesn't know the disquietude warring inside of her that keeps her from fully giving herself over to him. He licks her until her legs shake and the cellulite in her thighs ripple in waves from his power. He pulls his face away and taps the nervous bundle of joy until it streams the liquid that lubricates his way inside of her.

His stroke is slow and determined, charting a new path through old waters. His moves are steady until she arches her back and lifts her breasts to the sky. Mosiah lays over her offered body and takes one nipple into his mouth. He is as attentive with her nipples as he was with her mouth and her mons. Kissing them, sucking them, drenching them until he tries to take a whole breast into his mouth. With his body he tries to devour hers. He claims her from the inside out. *Give in*, he demands of her. *Give it to me*, he commands her body. *Release just for me. Let me see all of you.*

Mosiah increases the pace of his stroke. Quick and successive. A steady, incessant tapping on a drum he can't see, but he knows is there. Jolene reaches for his waist. She directs his way to the call his instincts pump and pulse to answer. She lifts her own hips to give him more access, more leverage. Committed to the common goal she squeezes him from inside, hoping to wrench the pleasure out of them both. Moving her hands from his waist to her head, she pulls him to her. Face to face, fluttering eyes to fluttering eyes, she kisses him hard, long and strong, as their legs tangle and their bodies bump uglies.

Onto his back, she is upright on top of him, the cowgirl in the saddle. With her knees pressed into his sides, Jolene alternates from riding to bouncing, bouncing to riding, sliding up and down the length of his shaft with ease. He reaches for her breasts again. He squeezes, he massages, he kneads the tissue pliant and pliable under his nimble fingers.

Jolene leans over him changing the angle of their interconnection and giving him her breasts, once again, to suckle in his mouth. She bounces the heavy weight of her ass down on his body, playing her own drum, enticing him to make an offering. They rock and wave their bodies together.

Mosiah kisses, licks and sucks from breast to breast, his hands massage and cup around their sides like underwire. Jolene pushes her hands into his shoulders, digs her nails into his flesh, and kisses his forehead, his nose, his ears, his neck, and finally forces him to give her his mouth. She tongues him down as his hands find her waist once again. He lifts her and slams her down over and over until he violently comes inside of her. Jolene rides the wave of his ejaculation, quickening her bounces in search of her own release.

It eludes her.

She sighs her frustration into his mouth, working to kiss more life into her heated body. She expels his softening phallus, forgoing the deep relief she was searching for and settling for a quick payoff. Jolene rubs her exposed clit across the wet skin of his still throbbing dick until her body runs with a trickle of warmth that won't lead to the river of lust she hoped would emerge.

She sighs again, ends their kiss, and rolls off his body to lay beside him. Mosiah wraps one arm around her body and instinctively she curls into him. Her head on his chest, she listens for his heartbeat before the noise of the house interrupts their point of peace. He begins to lightly snore as he always does after they're done. Jolene lays beside him, listening until he wakes. She can hear the sounds of Sesame Street going off and Lydia crying for Toussaint to play another one.

"One more, one more," she hears Lydia whine.

"Stop, you're going to mess up my stuff," Toussaint yells.

Jolene closes her eyes tight and deeply exhales, thinking to herself, *This is not enough.*

2.

"C'mon, let's get in the shower," Mosiah says groggily.

He unwraps his arm from around Jolene and sits up in the sullied bed.

"Ugh, that's why my back was hurting," he says, pulling Jolene's black ink pen from where he laid.

He hands her the pen. She takes it from him and grabs her journal. She opens it to the place where she left off and puts it back inside without looking at the words she wrote. *Later,* she promises herself.

"C'mon, Jo," Mosiah says.

"I'm coming. I just have to pull this comforter off."

Jolene sets the journal beside the lamp on the nightstand and stands up from the bed. She pulls one corner of the peach and white bedspread and walks with it to the closet. She gathers it into the corner with Mosiah's work suit and her dresses, and then heads out to join him in the shower.

The water is hot by the time she gets in after using the bathroom, wrapping her hair, and securing her floral print shower cap. Mosiah stands with his back laid against the tile wall beneath the showerhead, his butt hovering over the faucet knobs for the tub. She stands in front of him, the water barely spraying her. With shower gloves on, Mosiah pours a dollop of the peppermint castile soap into his hands. He creates a lather immediately and reaches for Jolene.

With a heavy heave of her chest, she steps toward him. He turns her around and begins with her shoulders. He rubs his soapy, gloved hands onto her back and then works it in with his fingers, massaging and kneading as he goes across her back, down her spine, over her butt, and down to her legs. He squats down to wash her feet, running his fingers between her toes and rolling them around the spaces of his own hand like a master reflexologist.

"Mmmhmm," she lets out in surprised satisfaction. "You're too good to me," she says.

He really is, her subconscious echoes as she relaxes her feet into his masterful touch. *Jolene, you need to stop trippin'. How many men will do what he's done. Raise another man's son, give him his last name, dote on your little girl, start two businesses just to take care of the family, give you a massage, and call you beautiful even when you're thirty pounds heavier than when you first met.*

"Mmmhmm," Jolene moans again as Mosiah drops her second foot back to the slippery shower floor.

He works his hands up her legs soaping as he goes until he gets to her sacred space. He takes his time washing around it, cleaning the sides of her legs, making sure not to let the soap get to close to her opening, muffling his laughter as she moves from side to side from the tingling of the peppermint so close to her sex.

Mosiah stands up straight as he soaps over her belly down the middle of her chest and then finally each breast. He takes his time with each one, cleaning them as he loved them. He starts with the nipple, moves over the areola, and then into the depth of the skin protruding from her chest. Finally, he moves his soapy hands outward, around and under her breasts, cupping her body trying to feel what he thought he felt before. He performs his own exam, exhaling more and more as he goes, hoping to find indifference; no dents or dimples of note. Mosiah swipes his hands once more and takes off the gloves. He runs his face through the running water to clear what he knows is his look of consternation.

"You always were a breast man," Jolene says, shaking her head.

"I know," he says.

She pulls on the gloves, adds more soap, lathers, and performs the same routine on Mosiah. She washes his chest, his stomach, his legs, and is as careful with him as he was with her when it comes to caring for the extension of his masculinity. She laughs in return as he clinches the muscles of his legs when the peppermint soap gets to close to the split that leads to his inner workings. She washes his legs and feet, turns him around and makes her way up his legs, over his butt and across the wide expanse of his smooth, milk chocolate back.

Jolene kisses him in the middle, at the top of his soapy spine when she's done, and then holds her hands under the showerhead to rinse the soap away.

"You're all done, Love," she says.

"Thank you," he says.

Jolene pulls the gloves off of her hands, wrings them out, and shoves them beside the soap in the metal caddy hanging from the showerhead. She reaches her hand to turn the water off, but Mosiah stops her.

"Hold on," he says.

"C'mon, we gotta go. I gotta cook, it's getting late. Lydia should be in bed by now."

"Just hold on."

"What's going on, Mo?"

"Nothing. I just want to know how you're doing. You were dizzy not too long ago, remember?"

"You were right. The Spanx, the waist trainer, it was too much. I was just light-headed from not getting enough air."

"Are you sure?"

"I don't know what else would be wrong with me. What's wrong with you?"

Mosiah takes Jolene's wet hands and raises them above her head. Using his bare hands, he cups the tops of her breasts and works his hands down and around until he feels what he is looking for.

"Right here," Mosiah says. "You don't feel that?"

"Feel what? Just you poking me. I don't feel anything."

He takes her hands and makes her do the same thing he did. He guides her hands over and around her own body until he stops at the undermost side of her breast where skin dissolves into the rest of her abdomen.

"Right here," he says pushing her finger into her own body. "You don't feel that?" He also presses the same spot under her right breast. "You don't feel how it feels different from this side."

"No," she says.

Mosiah holds on to her hands and studies her face. *She's lying. She can feel it. She has to be able to feel that if I can.*

"C'mon, I'll show you," Mosiah says.

He turns off the water, pulls back the shower curtain over their clawfoot tub, and steps out onto the tile floor. Water drips from their bodies as he pulls her in front of the long horizontal mirror mounted above their double, deep set, square, marble sinks.

"Hold your arms up," he demands, standing behind her.

She lifts her arms barely above her shoulders.

"C'mon, Jo, lift your arms all the way up."

"Mo, I'm tired and I still have stuff to do. I have to cook dinner, get Lydia to bed, and clean up after those two downstairs, plus get my stuff together for work in the morning. I haven't graded my students tests, let alone started the lesson plan for the next few weeks. I don't have time for this."

"Yes, you do," Mosiah insists.

Jolene huffs as she raises her hands just above her head. Mosiah takes her hands and pulls them straight in the air, taking the bend out of each elbow. From behind he reaches one hand to the right breast and the other to the left. He lifts them both at the same time to expose the smooth skin beneath, typically hidden by the density of her mass.

"Now do you see what I'm talking about?" Mosiah asks earnestly.

"Not really," Jolene says, stepping forward until her naked body is pressed against the bathroom vanity.

"Look right here."

Mosiah drops her left breast. "You see, this spot right here," he says, pointing, "it's not on your left side."

"Okay, and?" Jolene says.

"And," Mosiah says, taking his hands away from her body.

How do I say this to her without freaking her out, but making her take me seriously?

"What is it, Mo?"

He pauses, then says, "I think you should get that looked at."

"For what?"

"Because I don't know what it is, and you don't either. You've never had a mole there, so I don't think it magically appeared overnight."

"You never know," Jolene brushes him off. "Besides, I was at the doctor a couple months ago. If it was serious they would have said something then."

She walks away from him, away from the mirror, and away from his concerns. *It's been there at least a week and it hasn't bothered me yet. I'm still functioning the way I'm supposed to. It's probably just something my body is trying to get out.*

Jolene stands in the bedroom pulling out joggers and a tank top from her dresser. Mosiah walks in and goes to the chest of drawers to retrieve his underwear, pajama pants, and a T-shirt. She doesn't attempt to speak to him. She ignores him; gathers her clothes and takes them back into the bathroom to dress. She rubs cocoa butter into her skin to reduce stretch marks, though it hasn't helped yet, and puts on deodorant before pulling on her clothes. She finally takes the shower cap off and readjusts her scarf to keep her hair smooth and straight while she sleeps. Jolene takes her time putting away the lotion and deodorant. She prolongs having another conversation with Mosiah by staring at her face in the mirror. She brushes and smooths her thick, but tweezed eyebrows with her fingers. Her touch lingers as she runs them down the sides of her light brown face, and across the darker circles beneath her eyes.

I look fine. I feel fine. He's worried about nothing.

"It's nothing," she says to herself, turning away from the mirror and leaving the bathroom.

She walks past Mosiah sitting on the sheeted bed. "I'm going to make dinner. Can you put a new comforter on the bed for me, please? There's one in the linen closet in the hallway."

"Jo, you need to get that checked out."

"For what? It's just a bump. It'll go away just like every other bump that appears on a random place on my body when I'm feeling stressed."

"This is not a random place, Jo. It may not be stress."

"It's nothing, Mo," Jolene reassures. "I would know if something was wrong. I mean, who knows my body better than I do?"

Me, Mosiah answers in his head. *I know every shape of you. Every curve, every line, every dent, dimple or piece of fat is mine.*

He says, "Just call the doctor, Jo. Have it checked out. If it's nothing, you were right, there's nothing to worry about, but at least find out for sure first."

"Fine, Mo. Fine," Jolene says, leaving him on the bed.

He's always worried about me like I can't take care of myself. Like I've never taken care of myself. I swear, between worrying and working, he's going to put himself into an early grave.

Jolene runs down the stairs to the first floor, holding her unrestrained breasts down with her hands. She pauses at the foot of the stairs to catch her breath. One hand gripping the post of the wooden banister, the other balanced across her chest, she waits for her air to regulate and the dizziness from the sudden movement to pass. She waits until she can stand upright and walk into the kitchen under her own power without alarming an overly protective Toussaint, or overly compassionate Lydia.

Her fingers creep beneath the hem of her tank top while she waits. She searches for what Mosiah was so concerned about, even during sex. The bump. As small as a butter bean, she finds it with ease. She squeezes it but it doesn't pop. It is firm and unyielding under her power. She smooths the skin from her two-finger grip, and drops her arms back down by her side.

Whatever it is, it works like a pressure point. So Amen for that.

"Mommy, I hungry," Lydia says as Jolene walks into the conjoined kitchen and living area.

"I know, Baby."

"I want something to eat."

"I know, Baby."

Jolene opens the freezer door. Lydia pushes her way through Jolene's legs to look inside. She asks, "Can I have ice cream?"

"You have to eat dinner first. It's late and you have to take a bath."

"Can I have a popsicle?"

"No, Baby."

"But, Mommy, I hungry."

"There are other things to eat besides ice cream and popsicles. How about some chicken and pasta?" Jolene says, pulling out a frozen skillet meal.

"Pasta and chicken is yucky." Lydia backs out of Jolene's legs.

"Toussaint likes it."

"TeeTee, you like that?"

"Yeah," Toussaint says.

"Can I draw with you?" Lydia asks, grabbing one of his papers.

"Stop," he yells, pushing her away. "I already told you I'm not drawing. I'm doing my homework."

He snatches the paper from Lydia and pushes her away from where he sits at the table. She falls to the ground and wails.

"Toussaint," Mosiah yells, coming into the kitchen. "You know better than that. She's four."

"She won't leave me alone. I'm trying to finish my homework."

"That doesn't mean you get to push around your little sister. You're fourteen years old. Act like it."

"Yes, sir," Toussaint mumbles.

"Lydia, come here," Mosiah says.

She scampers to him wiping tears from her eyes. Mosiah scoops Lydia into his arms, adjusts her on his waist and shoulder, and turns to Toussaint. He asks, "What's your name?"

Toussaint huffs out his disapproval. He gathers the papers strewn about on the rectangular, mango wood table, and shuffles them together.

"I asked you a question," Mosiah yells.

"I heard you," Toussaint says.

"You don't act like it. What is your name?"

"Toussaint."

"What is your full name?"

"Toussaint Tecumseh Walker."

"Okay then. Who were you named after?"

"Two great generals," Toussaint answers solemnly, used to the routine anytime he gets in trouble.

"And who are those generals?"

"Toussaint L'Ouverture and Tecumseh Sherman."

"And what did they do?"

"They saved people from bondage and oppression."

"And you have my name," Mosiah says, walking over to the table. "And who am I?"

"A Marine," Toussaint grumbles, shoving his papers under his arms.

"That means if you want to fight somebody in this house, your only option ever in this life is to fight me. You understand me?"

"Yeah."

"Excuse me?"

"Yes," Toussaint emphasizes.

"Now take your stuff upstairs, take a shower, and then you can come back down for dinner."

Toussaint runs with his books and papers to the stairs. Halfway up he stops and asks, "Mom, can I call my Dad after dinner?"

Jolene looks to where he stands on the steps, his body just out of her eyesight, and pauses before answering. She waits for him to come back down the stairs to see the disapproval in her eyes.

"Can I, Mom?" Toussaint asks, ducking his head down to see Jolene in the kitchen.

"For what, Toussaint?" Jolene asks.

"To see if I can go to his house this weekend."

"Yeah, you can call him," Mosiah answers.

"Mom?"

"Yes, Toussaint," Jolene answers. "Now go on."

Toussaint runs the rest of the way upstairs. They can hear the sound of his feet going from his room to the bathroom above their heads.

"You know he's only asking to go see Jemarcus because you yelled at him," Jolene says, stirring the food in the skillet.

"I know. But it's not like we can tell him 'No, you can't call your Dad every time you get mad.' He wants to call, let him call."

"So he can get his hopes up just to be disappointed again?"

"Jemarcus has been more consistent lately . . . you never know," Mosiah says. "Hey sleepyhead." Mosiah tickles Lydia under her chin.

"Daddy, stop," she ekes out between giggles.

"You're getting too heavy for Daddy," he says, setting her back down on the floor. "Go lay down on the couch until Mommy calls you to eat."

"Mo, can you give her a bath for me, please. Dinner will be done in a second."

"Yeah. C'mon, Baby Girl. Come take a bath."

Lydia rolls her body off of the beige couch and runs back to Mosiah. He picks her up and carries her upstairs. It isn't long before Jolene hears water running in both upstairs bathrooms; their master, and the bathroom Lydia and Toussaint will eventually share.

She stirs the frozen pasta and chicken to life in the cast iron skillet given to her as a wedding present by her grandmother. Her grandmother who bought her the entire Williams Sonoma cast-iron cookware set as their wedding gift. In the card she taped to the box, she scrawled "You're finally doing it right. I'm proud to watch you get your life on track. Love, Granny Mae." The message, a not so subtle dig at how her entire family wrote her off when she popped up pregnant at sixteen.

Early in the summer after her junior year, she broke the news to Jemarcus and then, her mother and father. Her grandmother, Mae Ellen Lewis, found out shortly thereafter. For her devoutly Christian grandmother, an abortion was not an option, and so she promised to keep Jolene's baby, as long as Jolene didn't throw her life away. A decision Jemarcus nor his parents were none too happy about.

Jolene had her baby and named him Toussaint, after the general she never learned about in school. She picked the name from a book of poems that had a black girl in an orange do-rag on the front cover. His middle name, Tecumseh, from her favorite lesson in history class when she finally did learn about the civil war, or as the teacher called it, "The war of Northern Aggression." A man who burned through the South to free slaves, restore the union, and prove a point, was a man that was all right with her. His last name had been Lewis until Mosiah insisted on adopting him after they were married, and Jemarcus didn't protest.

"Jemarcus," she says out loud.

Jolene turns the heat down beneath the skillet and covers it with a plate. She walks to the counter top behind her where her phone is plugged in, and picks it up. Opening her messages, she texts him:

Toussaint is going to call you in a little while. He wants to come over this weekend.

Jolene sends the heads up and closes her messages, knowing good and well she won't get a response back. *I'll be lucky if he answers the phone when Toussaint calls.* Jolene puts the phone on do not disturb and leaves it on the counter. It will stay there until the alarm goes off in the morning and she's forced to get out of the bed, come downstairs, and turn it off. It keeps her from hitting the snooze button until the last minute, and then rushing everybody to get up and get dressed and get to school. The phone is also plugged in right beside the coffee pot, making her morning routine that much easier. Phone off, coffee on. She doesn't go back upstairs until after she's drank at least half of her first cup.

Jolene moves around the kitchen trying to keep her mind off of her body. *I should set a reminder to call the doctor in the morning, so I don't forget.* The thought comes and goes as she gets a carton of chicken stock out of the pantry. Back at the stove, she lifts the plate and sees the food is drying out and starting to stick to the bottom of the nonstick pan. She added water at first like the directions on the back of the bag called for. Now she pours some of the chicken stock into the pan to add more flavor.

"It smells good down here," Mosiah says, coming back down the stairs.

"Dinner is ready," Jolene says.

"Mommy, I wanna eat," Lydia says, sitting on the long bench on the side of the table for her and Toussaint.

"I'm fixing your plate right now," Jolene says.

"Did you make the garlic bread?" Mosiah asks.

"I didn't. If you want it, you can get it out the freezer. If you put it in the toaster it won't take long."

"Alright."

"Where is Toussaint?"

"Still upstairs in his room," Mosiah says.

"That boy knows he can catch an attitude," Jolene says. "Just like his damn daddy."

"Mommy, don't say that," Lydia scolds.

"I'm sorry, Baby. Here's your food." Jolene places a small plate in front of her daughter. "Do you have your fork?"

"No. I forgot."

"Then get down and get your fork and you can eat after you say grace," Jolene directs. "Mo, how much do you want?"

"Make your plate first. I'll get what's left," Mosiah says.

"I'm not that hungry and I need to be doing some schoolwork. These two are for you and Toussaint."

She sets the plates down and moves through the living room toward the stairs at the front of the house.

"Mommy, can I have some juice?" Lydia asks.

"You can have some water," Mosiah answers.

"Daddy, I don't want water."

"Or you can have nothing."

Jolene doesn't hear Lydia's protest as she goes upstairs. She walks to the far end of the hall and opens the door to Toussaint's room.

"Come eat," she says, peeking her head in the door.

Inside she sees Toussaint standing in front of his dresser, a towel wrapped around his waist, applying lotion to his chest.

"I'm coming," he says, not turning around.

"What are you doing?" Jolene asks, coming further into the room.

"I'm talking to my dad," Toussaint says, pointing to the phone on the dresser.

Jolene stills her body and says, "Hi, Jemarcus."

"Hey, Jo," she hears through the phones speakers.

"Toussaint, when you finish on the phone with your dad go downstairs and eat."

"I will."

"And make sure you clean my kitchen when y'all finish."

He huffs, "Yes, ma'am."

Jolene backs out of the room and closes the door on Toussaint flexing in front of the mirror, looking every bit like the Jemarcus she met in middle school. He was the new boy in their eighth grade class. He and his family had recently moved to a different neighborhood and so he had to go to a different school. She remembers he walked in wearing jeans and a wrinkled, short sleeved button down white shirt, and sat right beside her, since his last name was Lenard and hers was Lewis. She introduced herself and offered to show him around since he didn't know anybody. He agreed, and she smiled to herself because she had first dibs on the new cute boy all the girls in the class were talking about that morning in the courtyard.

Jemarcus had a tan skin tone with wooly brown hair, light, sleepy eyes, a wide nose, and a heavy bottom lip. He and Jolene became friends immediately, much to Mosiah's chagrin. He'd known Jolene since pre-school. They'd always gone to the same school and were typically in the same class. He lived at one end of the block in their Arlington neighborhood and she lived at the other. Back then, Jolene wasn't interested in Mosiah. Jemarcus was new. New to the neighborhood. New to the school. New to look at. Their friendship progressed from middle school to high school, and at 16, when she was finally allowed to date, the school boyfriend she hid from her parents, she finally brought home for them to meet. She gave Jemarcus her virginity, the same day he met her family, in the back of his beat-up Pontiac Grand Am.

The back seat of his Pontiac, parked beneath a large tree, in a secluded historic park near the river became her favorite place to be. Away from her parents, away from her sisters, away from Mosiah. She and Jemarcus had sex like they discovered it through the end of their school year, and into the hazy hot summer, until Jolene realized she was two periods late, and life as she knew it was over.

Granny Mae's decision was final, Jolene started showing and Jemarcus ditched her for a girl named Franchesca, who was a year younger than them. Mosiah, however, was still around. He picked her up for school when Jemarcus stopped. He carried her book bag so she wouldn't strain her back, and came to the hospital after she delivered, all dressed up in his rented tux from prom. He was still her friend through it all. He even wrote her a few letters when he went away to the Marine Corps.

Jolene made good on her promise to her grandmother and graduated high school and college with Toussaint in tow. It was a week before her college graduation when she realized Mosiah had come home from the Corps. She found him by accident when she was looking for a barbershop to take Toussaint after Jemarcus had flaked on her again. She walked in to the shop off Fort Caroline Road that said "Walk-ins Welcome" on the front, and there he was in the empty shop. It wasn't until later she realized Mosiah was the "Mo" from the sign on the door that said *Mo's Precision Cuts*.

She ran into him that day and she's been with him ever since. Mosiah, not Jemarcus, came to her graduation. He cut Toussaint's hair, and even cut her own hair when she got tired of growing out her relaxer and decided to big chop. He courted her, took her on dates, played with Toussaint, and proposed with the blessing of her parents and Granny Mae. By the time Lydia was born, looking just like Jolene, he'd already adopted Toussaint and no one ever questioned who belonged to who in the family made up of several shades of brown.

He's been nothing but good to me.

It is the only thing Jolene can bring herself to write in her journal entry that began with her despondence. She doesn't scratch out her earlier words. A promise she made to herself when she first started journaling. "Leave everything there, even if you disagree with yourself later," she told herself.

Sitting in the bed beneath the covers with her journal in her lap and her pen in hand, Jolene reads over what she wrote before continuing her new line of thought.

He's been nothing but good to me, but could he be better? Could we be better? Or maybe better is not the right word. Could we be more exciting. More adventurous. We act like we're old. We don't do anything. We don't go anywhere. He works and then he works some more. I work, and go to school. I swear this masters is going to kill me. I told Granny Mae I was going to get it for her, but they may have to roll my coffin across the stage the way these professors like to assign work. I hope they realize people choose online school because it's supposed to be easier. But with all their assignments, I hardly assign work to my own classes. Ain't nobody got time to be doing homework and then grading homework, too. As long as the kids pass their FSA and I get a good evaluation, I'll get my bonus. Then maybe we can take a vacation. That would be nice. We can take the kids to the Bahamas or something. Damn, Lydia doesn't have a passport yet. I guess I'll just add that to my list of things to do. That reminds me, I have to go by and see Momma and Daddy tomorrow. They say Granny Mae isn't doing too good and I'm sure my crazy ass sisters aren't helping. To be the one everybody wrote off for having a baby, they sure as hell don't have their shit together. But who am I kidding, I barely have my own life together. And Mosiah walks around here like he don't have a care in the world. Just cutting hair and cleaning buildings. Day in and day out. He doesn't ask for more. He doesn't even seem like he wants more. So much for him working so much, so that we can have whatever we want. He doesn't like buying anything. Well, that's not true. He doesn't mind buying. He just doesn't like shopping. Hell, who does? Maybe that's why we don't get anything, because I don't like shopping either. The only person that ever asks for anything is Lydia, and Toussaint gets stuff before he even thinks he needs or wants it. I love that he overcompensates so Toussaint doesn't feel left out, but I wish he had other dreams, other goals besides just being the rock of the family and providing. Maybe he does have other aspirations in life, and I just don't know about them. And if that's true, then that's the problem, because from where I'm sitting, it looks like he's just content to live a regular, unspectacular life, and die. For me, that's just not enough. It's not enough.

Jolene pulls open the drawer of the night stand and puts her pen inside. She stretches the attached leather cord into the journal to keep her place, sets it beside the pen, and closes the drawer.

I should be doing some homework since I've got some quiet time. But I'm not.

Jolene slides her body down into the bed and closes her eyes, even though she's not tired. The dizziness is gone, the shortness of breath she felt when Mosiah pulled her from the bed is gone. She lays there on her side, looking toward the windows covered by closed blinds, and sheer curtains. The sun has long gone down. One hand under her cheek, the other beneath her tank top, her fingers move over her belly and under her breast until she finds the bump in the road on her body. She pulls and squeezes the solid mass until her skin around the bump is sore and drowsiness sets in. She lets herself go and promises on the periphery of sleep to call the doctor in the morning.

3.

"When you finish your test, bring it to my desk and place it in the in basket," Jolene says in front of the class. "If it's not in the basket. That means I didn't get it, and you will get an F, no questions asked, and no excuses given. Do you understand?"

Jolene's class grumbles various versions of "yes" as they begin their test. It is the first in a series of practice tests she will give over the next few weeks to prepare them for the comprehensive end of course exam that will take them from Native Americans's America, all the way through the constitution and the amendments, with special bonus questions at the end focusing on her extra slavery lessons she gave over the course of the year. The practice tests were also her way of gauging her students progress without making them do homework. She grades the tests as they turn them in, so she doesn't have to take them home herself.

Jolene sits behind her desk in one of the few classrooms that is actually inside a main school building and not in a portable. She logs in to the school-issued computer and surfs away from school district related sites. She heads to Blackboard to look at the assignments and discussion questions she told herself she would complete and answer the night before in her online master's program at Florida International University. Looking at the list of overachievers who turned in homework papers, and left enough comments on posts, they ended up arguing with their own ideas and opinions, overwhelms her before she even begins. She closes the site, sits back in the hard, wooden desk chair she had to overlay with body cushions and pillows to make it comfortable, and waits for her students to finish their tests.

She reclines her neck back on the chair and closes her eyes. Her hands find her body. Instinctively, they work to feel beneath the fabric to the layers of skin. She pokes and presses the pads of her fingers into her tight white T-shirt, searching for the newly discovered bump beneath her breasts.

Her search is futile, the constant stabbing at her chest unnecessary. Her fingers rebound away from her body, repelled by the layers of cloth playing keep away. The t-shirt, the waist trainer, the Spanx, her bra, all provide a fortified fortress around the bump she didn't identify, and Mosiah hounded her to recognize.

I'll call the doctor when school is over.

Jolene sits up in the chair and opens her eyes. The first student comes forward, places the test in the basket, and walks back to their desk. She picks up the test and her red Sharpie and begins to mark through the test. She made the practice exam a mixture of multiple choice, fill in the blanks, and matching exercises that would even help the the kid who didn't do the reading, as long as they used common sense. She designed her class and her lesson plans to be easy to grasp and understand, knowing school was hard enough with ever changing standards, applications, and equations for how to do math, and speak the Queen's English.

Jolene reads through the first test. She writes 100 on the paper, and then shakes the mouse on her computer to input the number into her digital grade book. More students come forward, mostly girls, and then a few boys. Jolene knows her stragglers. The ones who will look at the test until the bell rings, and then decide to try to fill in a few blanks, and ask if they can stay late to finish. They don't know it yet, but today she has declined their request.

I have things to do after school. I have to get Lydia from daycare, Toussaint from school, stop by and see Mama, Daddy, and Granny Mae, and then there's today's extra choir rehearsal. Today is not the day to stay late and play at school. Hell, I have my own damn school work to do.

Jolene stands up from her chair and says, "The bell is going to ring in five minutes. I suggest those of you who are still working get finished so we can all go home on time."

Murmurs rise in the room among those who are done as they wait for those who are not to finish. Jolene hears snatches of conversations about video games, and who to follow on Insta and Snap, even though none of the girls talking are old enough to truthfully be on the popular social media sites. She listens as a few girls talk about getting manicures, pedicures, and facials at a birthday party for another classmate, that was held at a spa that caters specifically to children.

Lord knows what's going to be around when Lydia gets to be their age. If Tanya, Vaughn and I had half as much as these girls have today, I don't think we would have known what to do with ourselves. I hope they're at the house when I stop by to see everybody. That way, I don't have to make no extra trips to see somebody we missed on the first go round.

Brrrr-ing. Brrrr-ing. Brrrr-ing.

The bell sounds and the students who finished their tests hop out of their seats first, running into the coat closet to retrieve their book bags and maybe an umbrella.

"That's the bell," Jolene calls out to the three students still working on the test. "Finish the question you're on and turn it in now."

The three boys furiously scribbling and scratching on their papers, stand up and walk to Jolene's desk, one by one. With lowered heads and solemn faces, they place their test papers into her in basket and walk off to the coat closet. Jolene grabs the test from the hand of the last student, a young boy with unruly hair that is neither an afro, or dreadlocks, twists or braids.

"Did you study, Danté?" Jolene asks.

"Lil' bit," he answers.

"How about next time you do a little more than a 'lil bit." Jolene suggests.

"A'ight, Mrs. Walker. A'ight."

"We're going to do this again next Friday, so be ready."

"The same test?"

"Now why would we do the same thing we did this Friday, next Friday. Time moves forward. We can only learn from our past."

"I know, Mrs. Walker, I know."

"Then act like you know. Go on get your stuff so you don't miss your bus. I'll see you Monday."

Danté is in and out of the coat closet in a matter of seconds. A small backpack is slung across his shoulders. He walks with a light bop, tugging at the corners of his shirt, massive head phones are on his head, and a phone is in his hand. Jolene grabs her purse and her laptop bag and follows him out of the door.

She watches as Danté disappears into the crowd of dismissing children heading for the front doors to either get on school buses or be corralled in parent pick-up lines. A line similar to the one she will wait in for Toussaint when his school lets out in an hour. Before picking him up, she heads to the teacher's lounge to steal the thirty minutes of peace she has found for herself in a life filled mostly with other people's children and their drama, along with her own family. In the dark, windowless room, Jolene passes by the other fifth grade teacher, and one of the kindergarten teachers. They are huddled together, side by side, at one of the tables. Jolene waves her greeting and keeps moving to the little love seat in the corner of the room. She sets her purse and bag on the floor and falls into the cushions of the small, leather sofa. She feels her layers of shape wear collapse in on her body from her flopping down in the seat. Jolene resists the urge to unbutton the top button of her black jeans. She, instead, leans her head against the wall and listens to herself breathe.

The stuffy teacher's lounge, with its persistent smell of stale coffee and burnt popcorn, is the closest she can get to a meditation room or prayer closet. Hearing the clock tick, the last of the school bells ring, and other people's conversations, is the closest she can find to total silence, aside from the few moments she's able to steal away with her journal at home. But even that time is interrupted with the constant listening of Lydia crying, Toussaint complaining, or Mosiah scolding, disciplining, and complaining. At home she is forced to be Jolene the wife, or Jolene the mother. At school she takes on the role of Jolene the teacher. She is by reason of her birth, Jolene the daughter, and because of her faith, Jolene the servant; serving on the first connections team, teaching Sunday school, vacation bible school, and singing in the choir. There is only one time in her day, and one place in her life where she can just be Jolene Marie Lewis Walker. Not the teen mother who turned her life around, or the woman everyone looks up to because she seems to have it all together. In the teacher's lounge, for thirty minutes, she can finally be herself. If she needs to cry, sometimes she does, if she wants to write, sometimes she does. Her journal is always packed in her purse every morning, and put back in her nightstand every evening. For now, though, she leans her head against the wall, with her eyes closed, and breathes.

The smell of the coffee and popcorn is a pleasing aroma to her because it means she's by herself, even if she's not truly alone. The sound of the clock gives her something to concentrate on to clear her mind, and keep the time until her own alarm goes off to remind her to leave her comfort zone and return to real life to get Toussaint from school. She ignores the teachers' voices in the background. She owes her colleagues nothing, not even her kindness and cordiality. She sits in her corner, having waved to them so as to not be rude, and waits for her rude awakening. The alarm telling her she must return to the real world, to the people who depend on her, to the people who need her, to the people who look up to her, to the people who want something from her.

She waits, eyes closed, breath shallow, heartbeat slowing, and ears open.

"I'm leaving after this school year," Jolene hears the kindergarten teacher say.

"But why?" The other fifth grade teacher demands to know. He reasons, "You can do social work here."

"Because there's nothing for me here," she says. "I'm not even from here. I came with Teach for America to get my loans paid off, and then I stayed because I thought Jacksonville wasn't so bad. And we know how that all ended."

"Yeah, but now it's all over. I mean, it's been three years."

"And it'll really be over once I move."

Jolene clenches her eyes and her teeth, hoping to drown out the two voices getting louder around her. A woman wanting to run away and a man begging her to stay.

I wish I had the option to decide whether I was going to stay somewhere or just pick up and leave when I felt like it. I swear we lie to kids about life. Especially girls. We play house day in and day out, playing make believe at cooking dirt and leaves, putting dolls under our shirts pretending to be pregnant, taking care of the doll like it's a real baby, and driving Barbie cars and whatever else like we have real responsibilities. Nobody ever tells you as a kid when you have all that in real life, you can't just do whatever you want to do because it's fun. Hell, you can't go outside when you want to because it's usually work to do outside as much as there is inside.

Run, girl. You're single. Just leave. Take your life. Own your life. I wish I owned mine.

Jolene sighs deeply to herself and continues to rest. It is short-lived. The alarm on her phone goes off with blaring accuracy, urgency, and insistency. She struggles to sit up in the worn, comfy sofa, bend over and silence the phone, ringing from her purse. Hunched over her legs, the phone silenced, she feels a sense of vertigo. Her head is cloudy and spinning, her eyesight blurry, her shortness of breath from the night before returned.

Damn, I still need to call the doctor.

She waits, laying over her legs until any grasp of normalcy returns. Her movements are measured as she stands up from the sofa, holding the long straps of her bags. One by one, she slings her purse and then her computer case on her shoulders. She waits another moment before walking out of the teacher's lounge. A single hand, and a slight wave signals her goodbye to her two colleagues still arguing in intense hushed tones, over one's singular decision to leave the home and job she's made, in search of something better for herself.

Jolene takes her time walking the labyrinthine halls of the school, past classrooms and offices until she gets to the side door that takes teachers to their own personal parking lot, away from the hoopla of the children still waiting for a parent to pick them up, thirty minutes after the first school bell rang.

She chirps the alarm to her charcoal gray Kia Sorento and gets into the SUV in one motion, flinging her bags in the passenger seat. The inside of the car is scorching hot after sitting in the sun most of the day. It is the epitome of the maxim "hot as hell." Jolene starts the ignition. The AC on full power blasts hot air in her face and across her body. She turns the vents away from her, backs out of her space, and drives through the parking lot and into the streets of evening rush hour traffic. It will take her thirty minutes to get from Shady Grove Elementary school in their neighborhood, to the middle school all the way on the south end of the city near the St. Johns County line, where she knew Toussaint would get the best free education possible. But that's only in consistently moving traffic. Any hiccup: troopers patrolling the highway, drivers paying more attention to the construction work than the road, lost drivers, a blown tire, or a crash, and it will take her up to an hour to reach Toussaint, and then Lydia, who attends daycare in the same part of town. Thirty minutes to an hour in one direction, all to turn around and drive back to their neighborhood to stop by and see her family before choir rehearsal. Jolene breathes deeply as she merges into the highway traffic and prepares herself for the long commute, pleasantly surprised there are no slow downs.

She drives with lingering fog still clouding her head; the vertigo from the teacher's lounge not completely dissipated. She closes her eyes for a beat longer than a blink and opens them again, hoping to clear the remnants of shrouded dizziness. It doesn't relent until she's in the snaking parent pick-up line at Toussaint's middle school. She pulled in behind a line of other SUV's, mini-vans, and four door sedans at 4:40. Just late enough to give Toussaint enough time to play around with his friends in the hallway, before emerging from the school and running to get in the car.

"Hi, Mom," he says, slamming the door behind him.

"Hey. How was your day?" Jolene asks Toussaint as she pulls out of the school lot and onto the wide suburban streets of Jacksonville's southside.

"Good."

"What did you do?"

"Work."

"Obviously. What kind of work? What did you learn?"

"I don't know, just stuff."

"Do you have homework?"

"Yeah."

"Excuse me?"

"Yes," Toussaint corrects. He asks, "I can still go to my Dad's house today, right?"

"I have thing's to do, Toussaint. You can go as long as he's picking you up?"

"Oh. I thought you were dropping me off."

"You thought, or you told him I was dropping you off?"

"I … I told him," Toussaint says sheepishly, scrunching up his face.

"How nice of you to volunteer me for something you want to do. You could have at least asked me last night after you two got off the phone."

"I'm sorry, Mom. But can you please drop me off? Please?"

"I'll try. We have to stop by and see Granny Mae, at Mama and Daddy's, house before choir rehearsal."

Toussaint sucks his teeth. "Ugh, again," he whines. "We always go over there. And church too. Can't we just go home."

"If I thought you could watch your sister, then yes, I'd drop you both off at home; but since you can't be trusted to pay attention to her, or not fight, then you're coming with me."

"Mom, why can't you just take me home. I'm responsible."

Jolene laughs out loud. "Boy, for starters you're not responsible. And secondly, we have to pass Mama and Daddy's house before we even get to ours for me to drop you off. Ain't nobody got time to waste gas because you don't feel like being bothered. You don't have no wants."

"I hope Jovon and Riley are there," Toussaint says. "Man." He sucks his teeth, sighs heavily, and reclines the passenger seat of the SUV. Jolene laughs to herself as she pulls into the parking lot of Lydia's school.

"Lock the door. I'm going to get your sister. And don't change my radio station either."

"Okay," Toussaint says, laid back with his eyes closed.

Jolene hops down out of the SUV and walks quickly to the front door of the daycare center to get out of the dry spring heat. She signs in using her thumbprint and pass code, and walks the halls of the overpriced, state of the art facility where babies learn sign language, and all the kids do yoga.

Mosiah picked the upper-crust daycare center damn near in the next county since he takes Toussaint and Lydia to school in the morning, and has more flexible hours of when he opens up his barbershop. Jolene picks them up every afternoon. At Lydia's classroom she uses her thumb once again to unlock the door.

"Hey, mama's baby," Jolene says loudly over the music playing in the classroom as she walks in.

Lydia turns around from where she plays puppet master with a group of stuffed animals. She stands up with hands on her hips and says, "Mommy, I'm not a baby. I'm a big girl."

"Well, you're still *my b*aby," Jolene insists. "Come here, give me a hug. I haven't seen you all day."

Lydia runs into Jolene's arms. She reaches down to pick her up and squeezes her tight on the way up. She ignores the return of dizziness to her head as she works to steady herself with Lydia in her arms.

"Come on now. Mommy's gotta put you down. You're too heavy.

"I told you I was a big girl."

"I know. Get your bag and your things from your cubby, so we can go. We're going by to see Granny Mae."

"Will Mama Louise and Papa Rae be there too?"

"They should both be there."

"What about Aunty Tanya and Aunty Vaughn?"

"I don't know. If they're not there when we get there, they'll be on their way soon. Now c'mon, Baby, get your stuff."

"Okay. Okay," Lydia says.

Jolene watches her scamper off to the cubby with her picture on the front. Inside, Lydia pulls out her Barbie backpack. It falls to the floor along with six small dolls she had stuffed inside.

"I'm sorry, Mommy," Lydia says, looking up with pleading eyes.

"It's okay, Baby. Just put your dolls back in your bag so we can go."

"My papers too?"

"Get your papers too."

"Mommy, I made this for you," Lydia says, holding up two sheets of paper with a toddler's abstract art scribbled in rainbow colors across the front and back of the light blue construction paper.

"That's nice, Baby," Jolene says. "Now c'mon put it in your bag so we can go. Your brother's waiting in the car."

"Mommy, TeeTee hit me last night."

"I know. And he got in trouble for it, remember."

"No."

"Well, he did. Let's go."

Lydia shoves the dolls and papers into her bag and walks it over to Jolene. She hands it to her, before turning the knob to let them both out of the classroom door.

"See you Monday," Jolene says, waving to the teacher sitting in the corner of the class.

Three children fall into the lap of the woman with a glazed over look as the kids dance to sanitized, kid, friendly versions of popular songs blasting from the radio.

Jolene shakes her head on the way out thinking, *I teach, but this is a special kind of ministry right here.*

The teacher waves back, slightly delayed, as Jolene closes the door behind them. She switches Lydia's backpack to her left hand, takes her right hand, and walks them both past all the classrooms, the front desk, and through the security doors to the parking lot. Jolene knocks on the window for Toussaint to unlock the car and let them in.

"I can do my seatbelt by myself," Lydia announces.

Jolene waits until she straps herself in. Once the seatbelt clicks, she closes the back door and opens the driver's side. The AC is blowing cold. A welcome relief as Jolene sits in the driver's seat, feeling the sweat beading on her scalp underneath her still pressed hair. She closes her eyes to clear the dizziness once again. She presses her lids together, overcome by the heat she can feel, the sweat forming under her arms, and trickling from beneath her breasts down her sucked in, and restrained belly.

"Damn, it's hot," Jolene says aloud.

"Mommy, don't say that. Don't say damn. It's a bad word."

"Mommy's sorry," Jolene says opening her eyes. "But you don't say it either."

She turns around to glare at Lydia. The sudden whip of her neck clouds her head all over again. Jolene turns back slowly and grips the steering wheel to steady herself.

Something is not right. Now I have two things to call the doctor about. Well, one, really. Whatever that bump is will go away. Some people have back acne. Apparently I have chest acne.

Jolene backs out of the parking space, turns out of the lot and drives into the street traffic. She glances at the digital clock display of the SUV's smart system. The time reads 5:10.

Damn, it's too late to call now. Well, I can at least call and leave a message and follow up tomorrow. Yeah, I'll do that when I get to Mama and Daddy's house.

"Mama, Daddy, we're here," Jolene says, walking in the front door of her childhood home.

It is decorated the same as it was when she moved out and moved in with Mosiah to begin their new life. She walks into the three bedroom, two bathroom home and is immediately in the dusty dining room no one ever sits in. The mahogany dinner table for six is set with wedding china on top of embroidered doilies, cloth napkins folded like candlesticks, and all manner of utensils. It is the same setup her mother has for every major holiday when family and guests are actually allowed to sit and eat; otherwise it's uninhabited.

"We're in Granny Mae's room." Jolene hear's her mother call.

"Toussaint, go down in the living room or in the kitchen and start your homework," Jolene directs. "Call or text your dad to see what time he wants me to drop you off."

"Mommy, can I watch TV?" Lydia asks.

"Not right now. Toussaint has to do his homework. Come with me and say hi, to everybody."

Jolene drops her purse on one of the white cushions of the dining room chairs and moves toward the back of the house. Every wall she passes is filled with family pictures. Her parents' wedding day, baby pictures of her and her sisters, school pictures from kindergarten through college, pictures of distant aunts and cousins scattered across the city and throughout the country, and even a few framed obituaries of the dead are honored on the walls in collage picture frames.

Jolene walks into the back bedroom she used to share with her younger sister Vaughn. As the oldest of the three Lewis girls, she was forced to share a room when Tanya, the youngest, was born when Jolene was six and Vaughn was four. In the room the walls are white instead of the purple she and Vaughn settled on in their compromise of painting the walls red, Jolene's favorite color, or blue, Vaughn's favorite color. Instead of detached twin bunk beds there is a hospital bed with railings, a TV is mounted on the wall in the room that never had one before Granny Mae moved in, and the double desks she and Vaughn used to sit at to do their homework are now in her parents' garage, shoved in a corner with boxes on top and all around them.

The scent of camphor assaults Jolene's nose when she walks into the room. It covers the stench of the soiled diaper her parents just changed Granny Mae out of.

"Hey, Granny," Jolene says, standing by the entrance to the doorway. She resists the urge to hold her nose.

"Hey, Mama; hey, Daddy," she says, greeting her parents.

"JoJo, grab Mama's waist so we can get this diaper up over her hips, please," Jolene's father says to her.

Jolene walks over to the side of the bed where Granny Mae lays with her eyes closed and arms covering her face. Jolene knows she's not asleep. She knows her grandmother just closes her eyes when she has to be changed to avoid seeing her own son and daughter-in-law treat her like a child when she's the elder in the house.

"Mama, can I help?" Lydia asks, clinging to the back of Jolene's shirt.

"No, Baby," Jolene answers. "Stand by the door so you don't get in the way. It won't take us long."

Lydia follows Jolene's directions as she takes hold of Granny Mae's hips and waist.

"On three, Louise, you and JoJo lift and I'll slide the diaper up. Should take us two seconds. Okay. One, two, three."

Jolene remembers not to use too much force to lift Granny Mae. The last time she was called in to assist, she had lifted Granny Mae's light, frail body so high in the air she could have levitated for a moment if Jolene had let go.

The diaper goes on easily and Jolene sets Granny Mae's body back on the bed. Her mother and father walk out of the room as Jolene takes over. She pulls Granny Mae's duster down over her body, readjusts the blanket and sheets around her, then walks close to where she lays with her eyes closed. Jolene pulls Granny Mae's hands down, leans over her and kisses her on the forehead.

"How you doing, Granny?" she asks.

"I'm still living," she answers.

"You've got to be doing better than that."

"When you've lived a full life for eighty years, it's okay to just be alive now."

"If you say so, Granny."

"I do. Now, where's my great-grandbabies?"

"Lydia, come say high to Granny Mae."

Lydia runs from where she stands against the door post over to the bed. "Hey, Granny," she says with a grin.

"Hey, my baby," she says. "Where's your brother?"

"TeeTee is doing his homework in the living room."

"And what are you doing?"

"Talking to you. What are you doing, Granny?"

"I think I'm going to take a nap. I'm tired and I've been up all day."

"Can I lay down with you?" Lydia asks.

"Lydia, Granny Mae just said she was tired," Jolene says. "She doesn't want you in her bed if she's going to sleep."

"Uh, lil' girl," Granny Mae snaps at Jolene, "Let me decide who I do and don't want in my bed. Lydia, if you want to lay up here with Granny, then c'mon, Baby."

Lydia tries to climb in the bed. She stumbles trying, then turns to Jolene pleading with her eyes.

"Mama, help me," she demands in a trembling voice.

Jolene hoists Lydia into the bed and places her on the inside of Granny Mae's body, closest to the wall.

"You be quiet and let Granny Mae rest. You, hear me?"

"Yes, Mommy," Lydia says.

Jolene walks out of the bedroom and heads into the kitchen. Her mother is moving around the small space on the other side of the wall from the living room, pulling out ingredients from the refrigerator and freezer, the pantry and the cabinets. A small, circular table with four chairs is off to one side of the kitchen. It is covered with a white table cloth, and circular, straw place mats. It is the table she and her sisters ate dinner at when they were younger, while their mother and father alternated who would sit with the three girls if they were both home at the same time. More often than not, their father came in late and ate alone or with their mother, if she was still awake.

"Mama, what are you making?" Jolene asks.

"Just some spaghetti. It's quick and easy."

"You need any help?"

"Not with this I don't."

"Where's Daddy?"

"In the living room with Toussaint, helping him with his homework."

Jolene nods her head. She asks, "So what was the big fuss to get us to come over here?"

"Your grandmother was being difficult," she says. "You know how headstrong she is. She thinks she can do everything herself. And you can't tell her, her body doesn't work like it used to."

"You know she didn't want to move in here," Jolene says.

"We couldn't just let her live in her own house. It was getting rundown. She couldn't fix the little things that was wrong with it, and she didn't get enough in Social Security to hire somebody to do the work. It made more sense to sell her house and let her move in here."

"Mama, you and Daddy are getting up there, too, you know. How are you guys going to take care of her and take care of yourselves."

"I told your daddy that. But you know good and well that man is not going to put his mother in a home. You can forget that. When she goes, it will be right here in this house."

"Mama. Don't say that."

"Why not? It's true. We're all gonna go some time."

"I know," Jolene says quietly.

She drops the conversation on the one facet of life no one can truly prepare for, and that no one can explain. Jolene pulls out a chair at the kitchen table and sits down. She watches her mother move around the kitchen with a swift, determined focus.

Louise Renee Lewis, is short and thin, fair skinned, and has relaxed hair she's worn in a short cut since Jolene can remember. The opposite of her daughter whose complexion is a mix of her parents, with a body described as thick bordering on fat, depending upon the outfit and the observer, and long hair she keeps pressed straight, despite having gone natural.

Louise stands at the laminate counter beside the sink, and seasons the meat. Her hands move quickly from plastic jar to plastic jar, adding spices and herbs to the ground meat she insists on seasoning in a bowl, before dropping it into the oil lined pot to brown.

"Where are Tanya and Vaughn?" Jolene asks.

"I don't know. They were supposed to come over here after work, but they may not."

"Oh, Toussaint was looking forward to seeing Jovon and Riley."

"That's sweet of him to look out for his little cousins, even though he's so much older than them."

"He'd rather play with them than his sister," Jolene says. "Although today he said he wanted to go to his dad's house."

Louise rolls her eyes as she breaks up the browning meat in the pot. She runs her tongue over her teeth and says, "How is Jemarcus doing, anyway?"

"I don't know," Jolene answers to her mother's back. "Fine, I guess."

"Why does Toussaint all of a sudden want to go and see him?"

"Mosiah yelled at him yesterday for pushing Lydia around. He got his little feelings hurt, and you know how Mo is. He made him go through the thing with his name, and after that, Toussaint asked if he could go see Jemarcus."

"And Jemarcus responded?" Louise asks, turning around from the stove.

"Yeah, I know." Jolene says.

"Then maybe he's trying to finally be a father."

"I don't know why. He relinquished his rights and agreed to Mo adopting Toussaint as his own son. The only reason Toussaint has a relationship with him is because Mo insists on it, and I don't even know why."

"Because he's a good guy, Jolene," Louise answers, opening a jar of spaghetti sauce. "He's always been a good guy. You should know that by now."

"I do."

"Then I don't know why you're so surprised."

"I'm not."

"How are you two doing, anyway?" Louise asks.

"Me and Mo?" Jolene asks, her voice going half an octave higher.

"Who else would I be talking about?"

"We're fine, I guess."

"You don't sound fine."

"I am. Nothing's wrong. It's . . . It's just . . . Just . . . the same."

Here we go. This girl is never satisfied with anything, Louise thinks to herself.

She turns back to her pots. She nods her head and pulls a spoon out of a drawer, beneath the counter beside the stove, and stirs the sauce she poured over the meat until it's well blended. She keeps her skeptic comments to herself as she sets the metal spoon on the spoon rest, covers the pot with the glass top, and turns the fire down. Turning around from the stove, Louise wipes her hands against her black slacks. She's been retired from teaching for three years, but still insists on getting up everyday and putting on real clothes, even though she doesn't have anywhere to go.

"What's wrong with things being the same?" Louise asks.

"It's nothing wrong with being the same, but there's nothing wrong with a little excitement either," Jolene says.

"What do you mean, excitement?"

"Just what I said. Excitement. Something fun, adventurous, new, exciting. Something that takes my breath away."

"Jolene, stop living in a fantasy," Louise chastises. "You're married to a good man, you've got two children, one of them ain't even his, yet he loves him as his own, he runs two businesses, and has loved you since forever. If that's not exciting then I don't know what is."

"Mama, that's not exciting. That's life."

"A life you're blessed enough to live. Do you know how many women would kill to be in your shoes? How excited they would be to have a man like Mo?"

"So just because another woman would happily take my place, means I'm just supposed to be happy with what I have when I feel like I'm settling."

"Settling. How do you feel like you're settling? What do you want? Somebody like Jemarcus who didn't answer the phone, didn't come see his son, didn't contribute, didn't help out. He just didn't. Would his trifling ass be enough excitement for you?"

"Mama, that's not what I mean."

"Sounds to me like you don't know what you want."

"I know what I want."

"No you don't. If the only thing you can say is that you want excitement, then you don't know what you want. You're a married woman with children. All that excitement you're pining for is going to be wrapped up in these babies. Your life is not yours anymore. If you wanted to be excited then you should have kept your legs closed, instead of getting pregnant at sixteen."

"Mama, it's not like I planned it."

"I'm not saying you did. I'm saying you were reckless."

"What teenaged girl isn't?"

"So you mean to tell me when Lydia turns sixteen you will be okay if she comes home and tells you she's pregnant by some boy who doesn't care two shits about her?"

"Mama, no. I'd be furious."

"Okay then. Get your head out of the clouds, Jolene. We all have choices in this life. You chose Jemarcus, and then you chose Toussaint and yourself, and then you chose Mosiah. Now you have to keep choosing them every day. Find a different reason every day to keep choosing your family over and over again. Finding that reason, to truly choose the ones you love, I think is the most exciting thing of all."

"So why did you choose Daddy today? Jolene asks.

"I knew I was going to make spaghetti. I know he likes it. And when he eats it, he slurps just like a kid, and then ends up splattering sauce on the front of his shirt. He'll fuss at himself for it, but I love it because he enjoys the food that much that he gets his clothes dirty like a child."

"That's sweet."

"It is. But it's also exciting."

"If you say so."

"I do," Louise says. "Love is a privilege not everybody gets to experience. When you have it, hold on to it. It will be the most exciting adventure you can ever have."

If you say so.

Jolene doesn't say anything back to her mother. Still frustrated, she keeps her thoughts to herself. Her lightning rod of truth in her journal, the only expression of her true feelings. She gets up from the table as her mother pours the pasta into the boiling pot of water, sitting on the burner next to the simmering sauce. She walks back to the bedroom where she left Lydia with Granny Mae. Both of them are asleep. Jolene walks over to the bed and lifts Lydia into her arms. She hits the light as she walks out of the room and back toward the kitchen.

"Mama, we're going to go," Jolene says. "I need to get to choir rehearsal."

"Is she sleep?"

"Yes."

"Then you need to take that baby home and let her stay sleep. She go to choir rehearsal with you, she's gon' whine and fuss the whole time."

"I know. I still have to drop off Toussaint to Jemarcus, too and he hasn't even packed."

"Go on home then."

"I think I am. Lord knows I'm tired."

"Oh no, you want excitement. You can't be tired."

"Goodbye, Mama."

"Oh, don't get mad now. I told you, you got all the excitement you can handle right there in your arms."

Whatever.

Jolene walks out of the kitchen, down the short hall, and back into the dining room.

"Toussaint, get your stuff. We're getting ready to go."

"But Papa Rae is still helping me with my math homework."

"So do you want to stay with Papa Rae this weekend, or do you want to go to your daddy's house."

"I want to go see my dad."

"Then get your stuff. Take your homework to his house. He can help you."

"I'll do it myself," Toussaint says, gathering his books and papers.

"Or you can ask Mo," Jolene suggests.

"I can do it," Toussaint says.

"Suit yourself," Jolene answers. "Daddy, we're gone."

"You leaving already, JoJo?" He asks.

"Yeah. I'm tired and Toussaint still needs to pack for the weekend."

"Oh yeah," he says. "Where you going boy?"

"To my dad's house," Toussaint answers, swinging his book bag on his back.

Raenard Michael Lewis II doesn't say anything to Toussaint's proud response. Instead, he sets his deep brown eyes on Jolene. She stares at his dark face that is still chiseled with the angular cuts of his youth, despite his portly stomach. Their eyes play linguistic gymnastics, questioning and answering each other internally, instead of aloud, so that Toussaint does not hear his grandfather's dismay for his biological father.

Why's he going over there? Raenard asks his daughter with raised eyebrows.

Because he asked. Jolene answers back with a complacent look and shrugged shoulders.

What about Mo?

What about, Mo?

Okay, that's y'all business.

"Have a good weekend, Toussaint," Raenard says.

He crosses the living room and takes the three long steps that span the length from the front door to the opening into the hallway that leads to the kitchen. Jolene shifts Lydia to another shoulder and opens the front door.

"My sugar bug is knocked out," Raenard says behind Jolene.

"See you later, Daddy," Jolene says.

She turns around and kisses him on his cheek.

"C'mon, Toussaint," Jolene says stepping out the door.

Toussaint walks ahead of her to the SUV. Jolene chirps her alarm as another car pulls up in front of her. It is her sister Tanya driving her white Lexus. Jolene opens the back passenger door and loads Lydia into her booster seat.

"Hey, JoJo," Tanya says, getting out of her car.

"Hey, T," Jolene says.

"Is she the only person you see?"

The question comes from her sister Vaughn. Both Tanya and Vaughn were built like their mother; lithe and svelte. Only Jolene took after their father's side of the family of full-figured women, especially after having children, a shape she learned many men appreciated, including Mosiah.

"Well, I didn't see you in the car when Tanya was parking," Jolene says closing the door on Lydia in the back.

"I guess you're forgiven then," Vaughn says, coming to stand beside her sisters.

"You guess?" Jolene asks. "I don't need your forgiveness no way."

"Where are the kids?" Tanya asks.

"In the car," Jolene answers.

"Then let me say, Hi, to my babies."

"No ma'am," Jolene says, blocking the SUV doors with her body. "Lydia is sleep and you don't need to wake her up."

"Well, is it alright if I wave to Toussaint?"

"Be my guest."

"Hey, TeeTee," Vaughn says.

"Vaughn, the whole point of waving is so that you don't wake Lydia up," Jolene says.

"She can't hear me from out here," Vaughn says.

"Vaughn, the whole damn block can hear you," Tanya says.

"Whatever," Vaughn says. "Forget both of y'all."

"Why are y'all so late anyway?" Jolene asks.

"Vaughn," Tanya says.

"I should have known," Jolene says. "You never were known to be on time to anything. You'll probably be late for your own funeral."

"If it's as long as Aretha's was, you damn right I'ma be late. I don't care if I am dead, ain't nobody got time to be laying up there all that time, body turning colors and what not."

"You wrong for that." Tanya chuckles. "But it was a long ass funeral."

"Which is perfect for Vaughn since she don't go nowhere on time," Jolene says.

"It's not even like that," Vaughn says, defending herself. "I had to drop off Jovon and Riley to their daddy before coming over here, because I didn't know how long Mama and Daddy was going to need us."

Jolene was in her junior year of college and Vaughn in her freshman year, when Vaughn announced she was pregnant. Granny Mae made the same deal with Vaughn that she did with Jolene. "Finish school, and I will watch and care for your baby while you do." Just like Jolene finished high school, and then college, Vaughn had Jovon, then finished college with a degree in public relations. Shortly after graduation, Vaughn said she was pregnant again. Old enough and educated enough to go out and get a job, Granny Mae said her part of the deal was done, and Vaughn had to learn how to take care of herself and her babies by herself.

Vaughn got a job doing marketing and public relations for a non-profit, while Tanya, learning from the mistakes of both of her sisters, finished high school and college without any children. For that accomplishment her parents bought her a white Lexus, used, but it was new to her. Tanya's undergrad major was in business and finance. She now works on the investment side at a branch for one of the biggest banks in the country. Tanya took after their father, the accountant. Same jamocha color, angular face, and a love for numbers. Vaughn was closer in complexion to their mother, but put the three Lewis girls and their parents together and it was immediately obvious they were family. Captured at once they were the results of Mendel's laws of inheritance.

"So how's everything going in there?" Vaughn asks, nodding her head toward the house.

"Granny Mae was asleep when I left, and Mama's in there making spaghetti for dinner," Jolene says.

"Ooh, I wonder if she has garlic bread?" Tanya asks.

"I don't know," Jolene says. "Lydia conked out with Granny Mae, Daddy was helping Toussaint with his homework, and then me and Mama got into it."

"About what?" Tanya asks.

"My life. The same thing we've been fighting about since I was sixteen."

"So what's the problem this time," Vaughn asks.

"She doesn't understand why I want more from my relationship."

"What do you mean, *more*?" Vaughn asks.

"Just what I said. More. More than what I have now. More than what I'm getting now."

"Be specific," Tanya demands.

"Okay. I want more excitement. More adventure. More sex. More orgasms. More attention. More dates. More time for us."

"Jolene, you have two kids like I have two kids," Vaughn begins. "I'm not even married and I know sometimes all you have time for is a quickie, and a twelve pack from Chick-Fil-A."

"Then you should want more for yourself, too," Tanya says.

"Says the sister who hasn't ever been in a real relationship," Vaughn snipes.

"You don't know what I've been in."

"Is that right?"

"You can't hold water, Vaughn, so I know better than to tell you all my business."

"Guess you told me," Vaughn says.

Tanya rolls her eyes. "Anyway, Jolene, you've been with this man forever. Even when you guys weren't together it's like you were together. You're just in a place now where life is taking precedence over the relationship . . ."

"Okay, Iyanla," Vaughn says.

"But as long as you guys are together and still having sex — you are still having sex, right?" Tanya asks.

"Yeah," Jolene answers.

"Then I don't think there's anything to worry about," Tanya says. "As for that orgasm part. You better get yours, because you know he is going to get his."

"You could buy some toys too," Vaughn suggests.

"Oh my God. Could you be any louder?" Jolene asks.

"My bad."

"You know Toussaint and Lydia are sitting in the car."

"It's not like they can hear me," Vaughn says. "And they for damn sure don't know what we're talking about."

"Lydia's asleep, but Toussaint is not a little boy anymore. He might have his head phones on, but I'm sure his little nosy butt is soaking up every word. He's fourteen."

"Oh, so he has a little girlfriend now?" Tanya asks.

"I don't know, but last night I caught him flexing in the mirror after he took his shower."

"The boy just wants to look good," Vaughn says. "You know good and well he got that from his high-yellow ass daddy."

"Vaughn, you tried it. Jemarcus is not yellow. He's not even as light as you are."

"In the winter he is."

"Go in the house. Mama and Daddy been waiting on both of y'all."

"And I'ma tell 'em it's Vaughn's fault we're late," Tanya says.

"Whatever. They love me anyway," Vaughn says, walking toward the house set high up behind a grassy embankment.

With Vaughn out of earshot, Tanya asks, "Are you alright."

Jolene sighs, then says, "I will be. I'm just in a mood."

"What kind of mood is that?"

"One of those moods where all you want to do is listen to Mary J. Blige, Toni Braxton, and Meshell Ndegeocello because your man ain't shit and you don't know how to get out of the shit."

"Jolene, stop," Tanya says. "Mosiah is a good man. Better than most."

"I know. I'm just saying. That's the kind of mood I'm in."

"Well, you know Mary, Toni, and Meshell sing more than just sad love songs. You get the right Toni Braxton song and you might get pregnant."

"Yeah, it's not that kind of Toni song I'm in the mood for right now."

"Well, feel better," Tanya says, hugging Jolene.

"I will."

Jolene and Tanya, slow rock from side to side. She closes her eyes and exhales against her sister's neck.

"I love you, JoJo."

"I love you, too, T," Jolene says, letting go of Tanya.

She stumbles backward and bumps into the door of her SUV. Jolene holds the side mirror with one hand to steady herself.

"You okay?" Tanya asks.

"Yeah," Jolene answers. "Just got a little dizzy."

"Then maybe you need to come in the house and eat something with us."

"No, I'm alright. It'll pass."

"Okay," Tanya says. "I'll talk to you later."

Jolene watches as Tanya takes the sidewalk, and then the stone steps up to the front door. She holds on to the wrought iron banister for balance on the cracking, and chipping steps of her parents' house, the same as Jolene holds on to her SUV. Jolene doesn't move again until after Tanya has disappeared into the house and closed both the decorative storm door and the wooden door behind her.

"Mom, are you alright?" Toussaint asks as Jolene gets in the car.

"I'm fine. But thank you for asking."

Toussaint readjusts the headphones on his head, but keeps his eyes on Jolene. He is nearly unblinking until she turns the ignition and pulls away from the curb. Jolene doesn't look at her son staring at her; his usual heavy hooded eyes, alert and intense. She looks at the dashboard clock and sees the time coupled with the darkening sky all around them.

I still didn't call the doctor. I can just call tomorrow. Hopefully, Mo's not tripping.

Jolene sighs to herself as she maneuvers her way through the evening traffic. She turns the radio on to drown out Lydia's babbling now that she's awake, and provide a distraction from her own thoughts. Though it's no use. As her eyes jump from the palm and oak tree-lined street in front of her, to a discreet look at Toussaint through her periphery, to a look at Lydia in the back seat, bopping her head to the trap-laced R&B beat, her thoughts follow the same path.

Why did I even agree to let Toussaint go see Jemarcus during a weekday school night?

Because you need a break.

She answers her own question with the truth she's reluctant to admit.

I do need a break. But when am I supposed to take it. And what would I even do? I don't know the last time I've been to a spa. A massage is fine, but I hate getting a mani/pedi. The pedicure is not so bad, but by the time they get around to the manicure, I'm just waiting to be done so I can go back to my real life. I end up working myself into more anxiety, meaning the massage was a waste of money.

She talks herself in and out of relaxation until she gets to the corner and is forced to stop at the light. A CVS is to her right, a no name gas station with its detached convenience store, along with another food store are on her left. The latter is the lone business still in operation in the storefront lot with two vacancies.

"Mommy, can we get a snack?" Lydia asks.

"For what?" Jolene says.

"I hungry."

"Baby, we're a block from the house. You can get a snack when we get home.

"My daddy gets me a snack from the gas station."

"Well, I'm not your daddy."

Jolene makes a right when the light turns green, even though she could have made a right on red when she first pulled up.

"Mommy, can we go to the park?" Lydia asks.

"No."

"But why? It's right there."

"Because it's late," Jolene says, passing the park where a few children shriek, run, and scream across the jungle gym equipment.

"Man, I never get to do nothing." Lydia huffs.

Jolene turns her head to look at her, but decides against fussing at her.

She's just as frustrated as I am. That's life, baby girl. You don't always get what you want. Your life doesn't always turn out the way you want. I know mine sure didn't. It's not horrible. It's just not mine. Mama used to always say when I got pregnant with Toussaint how I was giving up my life. I didn't get it then. But it's true. The moment you get knocked up, your body, your life, the things you thought you wanted, no longer belong to you and no longer matter. Not for eighteen years at least.

I'm so glad Mosiah hasn't tripped out about wanting a son of his own, because I don't know if I'd be willing to do this again. Shitty diapers, crying babies, around the clock feedings. He was helpful when Lydia was born, but he was still gone most of the day. The fact mothers keep their babies alive is a miracle unto itself. I see why some wild animals eat their young. They probably just don't want to be bothered. I don't blame them.

Jolene sighs to herself as she blows through the light on Townsend Boulevard, passing another corner of convenience stores. She glances in her rearview mirror and sees Lydia looking out the window. Her chin is balanced on her fist, propped up by her elbow on her knee. Jolene opens her mouth to make a suggestion for the weekend, and closes it just as quickly.

Don't make plans you don't know if you're going to feel like following through with.

She adjusts her eyes back to the road as she makes a left into their subdivision and then a quick right into the driveway. With the car off, everyone moves on autopilot. Toussaint unfastens his seatbelt, flings the car door open, and jumps out in seemingly one smooth motion. Jolene takes her time gathering her bags and Lydia to go through the front door of the house. By the time she gets inside and closes the door behind her, all she can see is the light on beneath Toussaint's door.

She yells, "Toussaint, hurry up and pack your clothes so we can go meet your dad."

"You're home early," Mosiah says, walking to the door.

"I didn't go to choir rehearsal," Jolene says, answering the question he didn't ask.

"Why not?" Mosiah asks, taking Lydia out of Jolene's arms.

"Lydia fell asleep when we were over by Mama and Daddy, and I'm still pretty tired, so I called Ms. Helen in the car and told her I wasn't coming."

"I know she had a fit."

Mosiah walks over to the couch and lays Lydia across the cushion.

"You know she's too saved to say anything on the phone, or to my face for that matter, but she did tell me to make sure I knew my part or don't come on stage Sunday."

"I'm surprised she said that much," Mosiah says.

"She said it in her way," Jolene says sitting beside Mosiah.

"I'm sure. Did you call the doctor?"

"I didn't have time to. Every time I thought about it, I ended up doing something else.

"Jo."

"I know, Mosiah, I know. I have to take better care of myself."

"I wasn't even going to say that."

"I'm sorry. What were you going to say?"

"You need to call and see what it is? Has it gotten any bigger, is it leaking?"

"I don't know."

"You didn't check today?"

"Check what? How could I. It's not like I have time to get naked and do a breast exam at school. I'm teaching. The one moment I did have to myself these two teachers were in the lounge just yakking away."

"So you did have time to call, you just didn't," Mosiah says.

"Really, Mo. I have thirty minutes to myself a day. I've been tired. I've been dizzy. I've been achy and sore and I don't know why. Probably from sitting down too much. All I wanted to do when the bell rang was close my eyes before I had to go pick up Toussaint and Lydia."

"Jolene, if that's the case I can pick up Toussaint and Lydia."

"No. It's fine. You drop them off. I pick them up."

"Not if it's going to keep you from doing something important."

"It's not that important." Jolene stands up from the couch, walks into the kitchen, and opens the refrigerator.

I don't know why he's so concerned about this. It's one little bump. It's not like I haven't broken out before in weird places.

"Toussaint," she yells.

She hears the sound of running above her and then feet on the stairs, before he answers out of breath, "Yes."

"I thought I told you to clean my kitchen last night."

"I did."

"Not with this pot in the refrigerator, you didn't," she says, taking out a pitcher of water. "And what is all this stuff in the sink?"

"That's me, Jo," Mosiah says, coming into the kitchen. "I ate when I came home and just left it there. I was beat."

"Then, Toussaint, when you finish packing, make sure you come down here and clean my kitchen. Take the pot out of the refrigerator, put the pasta in the tupperware, and wash my pot. Then put the plates and stuff in the sink in the dishwasher."

"Ugh. Mom. My dad said he's ready to meet now."

"Then I suggest you call him back and tell him you're going to be late and that it's your fault."

"Ugh."

Jolene hears Toussaint stomping up the steps. She doesn't yell at him again for being disrespectful. *He needs to go see his dad this weekend. I need a break.* Jolene opens a cabinet above the kitchen sink, takes down a glass, and pours herself some water. She gulps the first and quickly pours a second. *I don't know what's gotten into that boy. It's going to be a long four years for high school, he keeps acting like this. He was such an easy baby. I guess this is my payback.*

"Jo, you alright?" Mosiah asks.

"Yeah, why?"

"That's your third glass of water."

"I'm thirsty. Probably dehydrated."

"You work inside."

"But I was standing outside talking to Tanya and Vaughn before I left from Mama and Daddy's house."

"You don't get dehydrated from ten minutes in the sun when it's going down."

How do you know what makes me dehydrated? Jolene cuts her eyes at Mosiah, but continues sipping her water.

"Did you tell your sisters or your mom what's going on with you?"

"No."

"Why not?"

"Because there's nothing to tell. There's nothing wrong with me."

"You don't know that."

"Mosiah, you find one little pimple and now all of a sudden you're a doctor who specializes in what's going wrong and right with my body."

"I don't need to be a doctor to know when something's off with you. I'm your husband."

"And I'm your wife. It's my body, and I would know if something is off. No one knows my body better than I do."

"Except me. I know every millimeter on you. You can't see yourself. I see you every day. Who would know what you can't see better than me?"

"Mosiah, there is nothing wrong with me."

"Then go to the doctor and prove me wrong."

"I will call them on Monday and make an appointment."

"We can go to urgent care right now."

Jolene cracks a smile. "It's not that serious."

"When it comes to you, to me, it's always *that* serious."

Well, damn.

"Boy stop playing," Jolene says blushing. "Toussaint, come on," she yells in the next breath.

Jolene pours her fourth glass of water and sets it down on the granite countertop beside the sink. She refills the now empty pitcher from the faucet that's fitted with a filter, and feeds directly into the water softener.

"I got it," Mosiah says, taking the pitcher from her.

She sips from her glass as he puts the pitcher away.

Maybe Mama's right. I need to get excited about the little things. The small choices that keep me coming home. He's always had good game. Even when I was too stuck on Jemarcus to see it.

"Toussaint, come on. The day is gone, and I don't have all night. You keep messing around up there and your dad will have to come and pick you up."

"I got it," Mosiah says, walking toward the stairs. "I'll get him, and I can take him to meet Jemarcus."

Jolene nods, "Okay."

He's too good for me to be feeling like this. But I still feel the same way.

4.

May 2

The last time I felt like this was before Mosiah and I got together. Toussaint was four, Jemarcus was doing what Jemarcus does best. Popping up for a week, disappearing for three. Popping up for a month, disappearing for six. No answers, no explanation, just a text or a phone call, or if he was really brazen and wrong, a knock on Mama and Daddy's door with his head hung low, his sleepy eyes peeking, and that lecherous smirk that always made me fall back in his arms, thinking he'd be there for us. I was finishing my degree and still stuck on stupid.

Even after I found out Mo was back and the whole haircut thing, I still wanted Jemarcus, even though he treated me like trash. But that's what I was used to, so that's what I came to expect for myself. At least that's what Doctor Fisher said. Now, what would she say? I'm finally doing well, in a relationship where I'm being treated well, living some woman's fantasy and I don't even want it.

What would Doctor Fisher say about me now?
Probably the same thing she always says.
"Happiness is temporary. What you're looking for is joy."

"Jolene," Doctor Fisher said in a slow, measured, observant voice. "Happiness is temporary. What you're looking for is joy."

Jolene sat on the the purple, paisley patterned couch with a wad of used tissues in her lap. Her tears flowed easily in Doctor Fisher's office since she was first officially introduced to the woman she'd only known in passing at the mega church they both attended.

Her mother and father invited Doctor Fisher to Sunday dinner two months earlier. An invitation that did not cause Jolene alarm. She was used to her parents extending invitations to eat to any of the two thousand plus members of the church, they happened to strike up a conversation with from one week to another.

That particular Sunday, Doctor Fisher joined Jolene, Tanya, and Vaughn at the dining room table with their mother and father. The gathering in the formal, front room was a rarity in and of itself. Louise didn't explain why she was setting serving dishes on the dining table, she only demanded that her girls pitch in. Dinner was casual and conversational. Over plates of rice, gravy, pork roast, roasted Brussel sprouts with bacon, and home made biscuits, the family and their guest discussed the sermon as much as politics and pop culture. Eventually, Tanya left the table to do homework and Vaughn was summoned away by the cries of a few months old Jovon. Tired of entertaining the overpowering estrogen in the room, Raenard slinked away to the garage he'd partially converted into his man cave, aside from all the storage boxes, to watch the football game in his recliner, drink a beer, and smoke a cigar. It was only then, when Jolene was left alone at the table with her mother and Doctor Fisher, that she realized Doctor Fisher was not an ordinary Sunday dinner guest. She realized she'd been setup for an intervention.

It started with her mother saying, "Jolene, did you know Doctor Fisher is a psychologist."

"No," Jolene answered.

"She is," Louise said. "If I had run into her a few years ago, I would have gotten you guys together sooner when you were trying to decide a major."

"Mama, you know I've always wanted to be a teacher," Jolene said.

"Well, psychology is a kind of teaching, right, Doctor Fisher?" Louise asked.

"In a way," Doctor Fisher answered tentatively. "If you look at life as a constant lesson, then in a way, my job as the teacher is to help instruct, or rather, guide my patients through it."

"See, it's teaching," Louise said, satisfied with herself.

Jolene sat at the table with her legs shaking and her feet tapping, praying, hoping Toussaint would wake up from his nap and call her name in need of something, anything to take her away from what she knew was going to become an awkward conversation. Her mother, still wore her nude stockings and plum-colored dress from church, with the thin belt at the waist. Her short hair was brushed and swirled to perfection as she smiled toothy grins, and preened, and fawned over Doctor Fisher while asking about the kinds of patients and cases she dealt with on a daily basis. Doctor Fisher regaled Louise with vague descriptions, and ambiguous scenarios of the patients in her practice she dealt with most often. Jolene caught on quickly that Doctor Fisher's specialty was in family and marital counseling.

The epiphany made her legs shake more, her knees knock, and her feet tap the time step, beneath the dining room table. She knew she was being setup and couldn't leave. There was nowhere for her to run. She looked first at her mother, who was laying the trap for her to fall into, and then to Doctor Fisher, the medium brown-skinned woman, with black, square-rimmed glasses, and salt and pepper hair pulled back into a low bun to show off the diamond studs sparkling in the two holes pierced in each of her ears. Jolene had seen her in church every now and again among the throngs of worshippers who came through the three sets of double doors into the long, rectangular worship center on Lone Star Road. From the times she'd seen her, Doctor Fisher had always been in a pants suit. This Sunday was no different. She wore tailored, black pants, and a sleeveless white, silk shirt that had long ties at the neck she crossed into a loose bow.

"Doctor Fisher, you know Jolene is going to graduate from Jacksonville University in a few weeks," Louise said.

"That's awesome," Doctor Fisher said. "You have a son, too, don't you?"

"Yes," Jolene answered. "He just turned four."

"That's amazing you still managed to go to school and finish, and take care of him at the same time."

"I couldn't have done it without my family," Jolene said. "Especially my grandmother. She keeps him on the days I have class or when I'm teaching at the school for my final credits."

"That's amazing," Doctor Fisher said.

"I don't know what it is about these girls of mine that made them want to be grown so fast and have babies so early," Louise said. "I about died when Jolene told me she was pregnant. And when Vaughn told me she was pregnant last year, I swear I had a mini stroke right back there in my kitchen."

"It happens," Doctor Fisher said. "But they seem like they're both doing well, handling it all."

"They wouldn't if it weren't for Mae Ellen. She's definitely their fairy godmother in the flesh."

"Well, thank God for her," Doctor Fisher said.

"I'm saying. I just hope Tanya don't get no notions of having babies from watching her sisters. After seeing how hard Rae and I work to provide for them, and make sure they have the best of everything, they just pissed it all away to be a baby mama."

"Mama," Jolene protested. "I'm graduating. I have a job. Toussaint and I will be fine."

"That's not the point," Louise said. "You're still a baby mama for that trifling, no good boy you keep running behind, who can't even keep his promise to get his son's hair cut."

"Mama!"

"Don't Mama, me," Louise continued. "You know I'm telling the truth. You've been walking around here looking cross-eyed and pitiful for days, and I'm tired of it, and you won't listen to me. Doctor Fisher, maybe you can talk some sense into her."

"I'm not sure what you want me to say," Doctor Fisher said, realizing she was as much a pawn in Louise's scheme as Jolene.

"Say whatever you would say to one of your clients, or patients, with the same issues."

"I don't have issues," Jolene said.

"We all have issues, Jolene," Louise said. "You just *think* you don't."

"Mama, I'm fine."

Jolene pushed her chair back from the dining room table, picked up her plate and carried it to the kitchen, fuming and mumbling under her breath the whole way.

Nothing is ever good enough for her. Toussaint is four. When is she going to get over the fact that I got pregnant in high school. I graduated. I'm about to graduate college and she's still at my neck. Daddy doesn't trip about it. She's so concerned about me and giving me all this grief, and she doesn't say anything to Vaughn.

Jolene pushed the door open to the bedroom she still shared with her sister and slammed it behind her.

"What's wrong with you?" Vaughn asked.

"Mama," Jolene answered.

She reached behind her back and began unzipping her yellow dress. Jolene worked the zipper to the middle of her back, near her bra strap, before she couldn't force it down anymore. Vaughn got and helped pull the zipper down the rest of the way.

"What happened now?" Vaughn asked.

"Mama just thinks she's so slick. She knew what she was doing when she invited Doctor Fisher over here."

"What was she doing?"

Vaughn sat back down on her bedspread and picked up the book she had set aside to help Jolene out of her dress. Jovon was asleep in the bassinet set up between their beds, where their night stand used to sit when they were kids, and before they had babies. Jolene, in just her bra and panties, plopped down on her own bed, careful to not disturb Toussaint. She watched him as he rolled over and yawned, but did not wake up.

Lowering her voice, Jolene said, "She set me up for an intervention."

"An intervention about what?" Vaughn asked.

"Jemarcus. Ugh."

"You need an intervention about him," Vaughn said, looking down at her book.

"Oh, so you were in on it too?"

"In on what? The intervention? No. But everybody in this family knows you need to stay away from him, but you."

"Well, thanks for telling me."

"Jolene, it's not like we haven't been trying to tell you since Toussaint was born and he couldn't even show up at the hospital."

"That's because of his parents."

"And that's why don't nobody say anything to you about it anymore. You always make an excuse for his behavior."

"And what about you and Emmanuel?" Jolene asked. "I'm not the only baby mama in the house."

"The difference between Jemarcus and Emmanuel is that Emmanuel comes to see Jovon. He came to the hospital, and he's here every other day to check on his son. When Jemarcus comes over, if he comes over, he only comes to the door. In all the years y'all have been dealing with each other, I don't think I've seen him come any further than the dining room."

"So that's what y'all do?" Jolene asked accusingly. "Talk about me behind my back every damn day, while I'm out busting my ass at school and at work trying to make sure I can take care of me and Toussaint, and not just be a baby mama."

She stood up from the bed wiping her eyes, as she tried to hide her reddening face behind her hands.

"That's the point, Jolene," Vaughn said. "You're out here busting your ass and Jemarcus ain't even trying. And yet you keep going back to him. The dick can't be that good."

"That's not even the point," Jolene said. "How about I just want us to be a family. I know I fucked up getting pregnant, but Jemarcus and I have been together since eighth grade. Y'all may say it doesn't count, but it does to me."

"JoJo, it's not that the time doesn't count, but what about now? You're not in eighth grade anymore. You're not in high school anymore. You're about to graduate from college and he's still doing the same dumb shit. You deserve better."

"I guess."

"No, I guess," Vaughn said. "That's all Mama is trying to show you with Doctor Fisher being here. That you deserve better. I guess she figures since she can't talk any sense into you, somebody else who doesn't know you, or us, or Jemarcus, can."

Jolene flopped back on the bed. Toussaint rolled over and opened his eyes.

"Hey, sleepyhead," Jolene said as he crawled into her lap. "You want to go to the library?"

Toussaint nodded his little head against her chest.

"Okay. Let mommy get dressed."

"And that's what you always do," Vaughn said. "Whenever somebody says something you don't like, you leave."

Jolene stood up from the bed. "I'm taking Toussaint to the library. I'll be back."

"I'm not tripping. Your beef is not with me or Mama for that matter. Whatever it is you don't want to talk about, or you don't want anybody to know about is between you and Jemarcus."

Jolene tossed the yellow dress she shimmied out of into the dirty clothes hamper in the closet she shared with Vaughn. She snatched a pair of jean shorts from a hanger, and grabbed a tank top from a pile of shirts on a shelf in the top of the closet. Jolene put both on quickly, and slid her feet into a pair of flip-flops.

"Come on, Toussaint, let's go," Jolene said.

Toussaint flipped his body off the bed and ran into Jolene's awaiting arms. She opened the door, marched to the front of the house, and opened the front door. "I'm gone," was the only thing she said to her mother and Tanya, who were sitting at the dining room table as she walked out.

Jolene stormed down the front steps of the house to where her car, a beat-up, old, brown Camry, was parked. She strapped Toussaint into his booster seat and got into the driver's seat. It wasn't until she was parked at the library, tears still streaming down her face, that she noticed the business card tucked beneath one of her windshield wipers. From the car she could read Doctor Fisher's phone number. Jolene called and left a sobbing message.

That message and Doctor Fisher's return phone call began her healing. She met Doctor Fisher every other week at her Jacksonville Beach office. A stone's throw away from the ocean, Jolene could smell the salty sea water in the air every time she traveled from her little enclave across the Intracoastal waterway. It was two months from their first meeting at her mother's house when Doctor Fisher first said her famous last words.

"Happiness is temporary. What you're looking for is joy."

"What do you mean?" Jolene asked, pulling yet another tissue from the box beside her.

"I mean, anything can make you happy," Doctor Fisher said. "Money can make you happy. Food can make you happy. Sex can make you happy. Even God can make you happy. But after awhile that happiness wears off."

"Okay," Jolene said. "So why doesn't joy wear off?"

"Because happiness is a feeling. Feelings come and go. Joy is a state of being. When you have joy you are intentional about it."

"And so how do I find joy?"

"You have to be willing to be okay with being hurt and feeling pain because you know it's good for you."

"That sounds counterproductive."

Jolene gathered the tissues surrounding her and balled them up into one giant wad of snot rags. She chucked them into a nearby waste basket and then looked Doctor Fisher squarely in the face. As always, her hair was pulled back, the diamond studs in her ears shined, and she wore a pants suit. Navy slacks, a matching blazer, a silk, teal blouse, and teal flats she had taken off to tuck her feet beneath her in her oversized, brown leather office chair.

Doctor Fisher said, "Being okay with the pain that Jemarcus doesn't want you is not counterproductive. It's exactly what you need to accept to get to your joy. When you have joy, you will let go of the things that are bad for you to maintain your inner peace."

"But who said Jemarcus doesn't want me?" Jolene asked.

"You did. In every scenario you've told me about for the last two months, his behavior screams that he doesn't want you with him. And guess what, he doesn't. The question is, why do you want him?"

Jolene was stumped and without an answer. She looked at Doctor Fisher and then switched her gaze to the decor in the room. Abstract paintings in earthy hues, Doctor Fisher's matted and framed degree from the University of Florida mounted on the wall, and a few encouraging Bible verses written in cursive on large wooden planks. Jolene focused on one that said "Count it all joy, my brothers, when you meet trials of various kinds."

Doctor Fisher turned to follow Jolene's gaze.

"Count it all joy, Jolene," Doctor Fisher said. "When you sacrifice the happiness in your hand to maintain the peace in your heart is when you know you have found joy."

Jolene nodded.

Doctor Fisher continued, "Try writing out your feelings in a journal. Being able to see them will make a difference in the intentions you set for your life. It will show you whether you are choosing happiness or choosing joy."

Jolene nodded her head again, less confused, but at a loss for words. She stood up from the couch because, whether or not her session was over, she was done talking. Doctor Fisher walked her from the office to the front door. She hugged Jolene and whispered in her ear, "Count it all joy."

Count it all joy.
Is Mosiah the happiness in my hand or the peace in my heart.

Jolene puts her pen in her journal, closes the book and sets it to the side.

I need to call Doctor Fisher, she thinks.

5.

"Jolene, come on in," Doctor Fisher says. "I was surprised to get your call."

"Thanks for taking me on such short notice," Jolene says.

She walks past the empty reception desk to the back of the small storefront building. Inside the last door on the right, Jolene turns into the office that says Dr. Antoinette Fisher on the name plate. The lights are off, the air is cool, and the scent of mint is heavy in the air. Jolene sets her purse on the floor and flops down on the couch. She pulls up her waist trainer, and Spanx beneath her shirt, to alleviate the pressure at her navel, where the button of her jeans keeps her sucked in.

"Wooh," she exhales.

"You alright?" Doctor Fisher asks.

"Yeah," Jolene answers. "I'm trying to at least look skinny, even if I can't be skinny."

"Good luck with that. So what brings you by today?" Doctor Fisher, asks sitting down in her chair.

Why am I here today?

Because my marriage is good, but it's not good enough for me. That sounds ridiculous.

Jolene moves her mouth from side to side. She stares at Doctor Fisher's serious face. The browning face only shows a few signs of age, a couple errant wrinkles, a misplaced mole or two, and cheeks just beginning to sag. Otherwise, Doctor Fisher looks the same as she did the day Louise staged Jolene's intervention, just in different clothes. Her hair is still pulled back in a low bun, and she wears tan slacks, a red V-neck blouse, and gold sandals. Jolene looks at Doctor Fisher and rethinks her decision to come.

Maybe this wasn't a good idea.

She is hesitant to explain why she called and asked to be scheduled for the first opening. She is embarrassed to say she jumped at the opportunity to take the Wednesday appointment at five in the evening, even though that meant making Mosiah believe she called a different type of doctor about the bump under her breast. That phone call, she has still yet to place.

It's not that big of a deal anyway. When I checked it this morning, it wasn't even that big.

"Jolene," Doctor Fisher says. "What's going on?"

"I think I want a divorce?" Jolene blurts out.

"Why?" Doctor Fisher asks.

"I don't know," Jolene says. "That's why I'm here."

"Did something happen?"

"Nothing happened."

"Then why do you want a divorce?"

"I don't even think I want a divorce." Jolene sighs.

Maybe I should have kept this to myself.

Jolene lays her elbows on her knees and lowers her head down. She breathes between her legs, stares at her purple painted toes, and counts to ten. She lifts her head and immediately, dizziness sets in. Jolene closes her eyes, exhales, and waits for it to pass.

"It's not that I want a divorce," she begins. "I just feel like everything is the same and it's not enough. Anymore."

"What's the same, and why isn't it enough?" Doctor Fisher asks.

"Our lives are the same. Day in and day out. It's the same routine. Get up, get dressed, make coffee, and breakfast, go to work, get the kids, come home, make dinner, get the kids ready for bed. Repeat. Even the weekends feel the same. Mo's biggest day at the shop is Saturday, and that comes off of his busiest day with the cleaning business, which is Friday night."

"Do you guys not get to see each other and that's why you feel overwhelmed?" Doctor Fisher asks.

"I don't feel overwhelmed. I just want something different." Jolene sighs. "You ever just wanted to run away from your life for awhile, so that you miss it enough to want to come back."

"We've all been there."

"Well, that's where I am now. I want to run away and see if I even miss what I'm leaving."

"Jolene," Doctor Fisher says, removing her glasses, "there's nothing wrong with feeling like you need an escape; some time to yourself. Have you told Mosiah how you're feeling?"

"No."

"Why not?"

"He won't understand."

"He definitely won't understand if you don't give him the chance to," Doctor Fisher says.

"I keep thinking about what you always say about being intentional about choosing joy."

"Yes."

"Last week I started to wonder if Mosiah is part of my joy or just temporary happiness."

"Jolene, you keep associating what you're supposed to have on your own with the things you can get from other people."

"But if I'm being intentional about being in this constant state of joy, shouldn't I examine if the things and the people around me add or subtract from this personal journey?"

"Yes, you are, but . . ."

"Then what's wrong with wondering where Mosiah fits into the journey?"

"There's nothing wrong with that, Jolene. But you don't wonder where Toussaint or Lydia fit into your journey to always choosing joy. It's only Mosiah you question," Doctor Fisher says. "Why is that?"

"If I knew the answer to that, I wouldn't be here."

"Is it because somewhere inside of you, you feel like you don't deserve him?"

"What makes you say that?"

"Because you said you felt that way even before you two got married. That he was your friend forever and you didn't see why he still wanted to be with you after so many years, and all that you put him through with Jemarcus."

"But we've been married six, going on seven, years now."

"And?"

"If I felt that way, I think it would have showed up before now."

"Not really," Doctor Fisher says. "You guys got married, and had Lydia, what, two years later? You never really had a honeymoon period to just be married because you already had Toussaint. These feelings may have always been there, but it seems like you haven't had the time to focus on them until now."

Jolene nods her head and runs through the years of their relationship. The reconnection at the barbershop. Her graduation. Getting a job, working, dating, engaged, married. She remembers the whirlwind of their wedding that they kept small because they couldn't afford anything big. They got married in his church, and had the reception at a small event venue just blocks away from the Arlington Expressway. Her mother and Granny Mae catered, and instead of a traditional cake, they had a cupcake tower for the few guests who were invited.

The day after their wedding was spent moving Jolene's stuff from her parents' house to the house she and Mosiah are in now. The one they saw was for sale when he was driving her home after a date. The first house in a tiny, block-long subdivision off Fort Caroline Road, Mosiah bought in a short sale. It was one of the cheapest houses on the block, with the homes in the culdesac costing upwards of a million dollars because the backyards were embankments that led to private docks stretched into the St. Johns River.

"At twenty-three I had everything I thought I ever wanted," Jolene says. "A husband who loved me and my son. A house and a job I loved."

"And now?"

"I still have all those things, but it just doesn't seem like enough."

"Why not?"

"I just don't feel like I'm growing. I feel stuck."

"Are you?"

"Am I what?"

"Are you stuck? Are you not growing? Are you not progressing?" Doctor Fisher presses.

"No. I'm in grad school now. We have Lydia. We've fixed up the house. Mo's opened another business to make sure we can take care of anything. So we're not the same as we were."

"Are you growing together in your relationship?"

"I believe so. I can tell him anything and he doesn't flinch. Hell, let him tell it, he'll say he knows me better than he knows himself."

"And you?" Doctor Fisher asks. "How well do you know Mosiah?"

"I've known him since I was kid. I know when he's mad even if he doesn't want to admit it. I know when he's frustrated, concerned, or when he's really excited, because that's when he starts stuttering because he can't get all his words out.

"Seems like you know a lot," Doctor Fisher says.

"Then why do I feel like this?"

"Because sometimes when life seems to be going too good, too well, we think that something is wrong. That we're supposed to have drama, because that means excitement and adventure. You have to remember there is nothing wrong with just coasting."

"I guess," Jolene says.

Doctor Fisher asks, "Would you like it better if you couldn't get Mosiah on the phone? If you had to follow him around because you didn't know if he was really working at the barbershop or not? Or maybe you'd prefer to find out he was having an affair and had a baby by someone else. Is that the kind of excitement and adventure you want?"

"Hell, no," Jolene says.

"Then be thankful to coast. I'm sure a million people would give you their excitement to just be boring."

"I know, but that still doesn't make me feel better."

"What's wrong with you is what happens in a lot of marriages. You get into the routine of life and you start to question everything, and wonder whether you can live the rest of your life like this."

"So you do know what I'm talking about."

"I never said I didn't," Doctor Fisher says. "My husband and I have been married almost thirty years. We've been where you are more times than I can count. Sometimes it was just me feeling that way, sometimes it was just him, sometimes it was the both of us together."

"So how did you get over it?"

"Sometimes we went on vacation together to just hit a reset. At other times he did something nice for me, or I did something nice for him. It's the little things that make you appreciate what's in front of you."

"Mama said something similar to me yesterday," Jolene admits.

"Really, what did she say?"

"She told me to remember why I chose him, and find a new reason to choose him everyday."

"Sounds like good advice to me. You should listen to Louise sometimes."

"I know."

"Now you do," Doctor Fisher says.

Jolene grabs her purse from the floor and unzips it. She pulls out the cash she took out of the ATM and hands it to Doctor Fisher.

"Thank you," Jolene says.

"Anytime."

Jolene stands up from the sofa and stumbles into the book case on the wall beside the couch.

"Are you alright?" Doctor Fisher asks, alarm written all over her face.

"I'm okay. I've just been having these dizzy spells every now and again. If I'm not dizzy, then I'm tired, achy, and super thirsty."

"That's a lot of symptoms," Doctor Fisher says. "Anything else going on?"

"No," Jolene says quickly.

She wipes imaginary dust from her arms and legs, then rubs her wrist she banged into the book case.

Doctor Fisher opens her office door, "If the dizziness and everything else continues, you should probably go see someone. Get a CT scan or an MRI just to make sure nothing else is going on."

The only thing is the pimple, but that's nothing. It's probably an ingrown hair. It was going down this morning. I might be able to pop it tonight and show Mo there's nothing to worry about.

"I don't think it's anything serious," Jolene says, stepping out of the office.

"Pay attention to what your body's trying to tell you," Doctor Fisher says.

"I will."

Jolene walks away from Doctor Fisher. She follows the white tile to the front of the building, past the reception desk that's still missing the receptionist, and out of the front doors into the hot sun. The smell of the ocean is heavy around her, and the sound of crashing waves is distinct amongst the evening traffic. Jolene inhales deeply before moving toward her car. She opens the doors, gets in, turns the ignition, and rolls the windows down. There's enough of a breeze for her to not need the air conditioning. She inhales the ocean air once more, throws the SUV in gear, and backs out of the space in front of Doctor Fisher's storefront office.

Maybe we need to move to the beach.

6.

"What did the doctor say?"

"She said pay attention to my body."

"What does that mean? What did she say about the bump?"

"I didn't ask her about the bump?"

"Why not? I thought that's why you were going to the doctor. The reason you needed me to pick up Toussaint and Lydia from school."

"I did go to the doctor. I saw Doctor Fisher."

"Jolene. You still haven't made an appointment to see a real doctor yet?"

"Doctor Fisher is a real doctor."

"You know what I mean, Jo."

Mosiah replays the argument he had with Jolene in his head as he snips tufts of the thick, wooly hair of the client sitting in his chair.

"Johnny, how low do you want it, man?" Mosiah asks.

"Low enough for me to impress these white folks at my job interview?"

"Oh yeah," Mosiah says. "Where you interviewing at?"

"Publix."

"Why you wanna work there?"

"I don't know, man," Johnny says. "I need a job."

"I told you, you could work for me."

"You don't pay enough here at the barbershop, and my moms says I can't stay out that late with you cleaning buildings, no way."

Mosiah stretches more pieces of Johnny's combed out locks to their full length and then snips them away until the teenaged boy in his chair begins to look more his own age, and less like a fourth member of the Migos.

Mosiah says, "Boy, you know good and well I wouldn't have you out late."

"It's alright, Mo," Johnny says. "Publix is good."

"I never said Publix wasn't good. I'm just saying, you ain't gon' be making no real money either."

"How much you pay your cleaning crew?" Johnny asks.

"My first timers start off at fifteen an hour," Mosiah says.

"That's not bad. How much you pay Leo to sweep up the hair around here?" Johnny asks.

"None of your damn business," Leo says from the back of the barbershop.

Eighteen-year-old Leonard Stokes walks from the back of the barbershop, pushing his broom the entire way. He keeps his eyes up, paying more attention to what may or may not come through the front door, than the hair and dust being picked up by his push broom on the black and white tile floor. His low cut hair, with deep, brush trained waves, shines with grease beneath the fluorescent lights. The end of a dust pan is shoved into the back of his tattered light wash jeans, and two gold chains hang from his cocoa brown neck, beneath his wrinkled, white, V-neck T-shirt. Leo stops in front of the red barber chair next to Mosiah's station. It's the only empty chair in the shop for six. Mosiah's space is in the center on the right side. There's a barber behind him, and three across from him. They man their stations behind a half wall that separates the service point from the waiting area, where customers rarely wait. Even still, it is furnished with a black futon, and a cheap coffee table where old issues of *Men's Health* and *Sports Illustrated* are scattered across the top. The walls of the shop are painted black with a high gloss finish; mirrors stretch the length of each. The barbers' licenses and credentials are matted and framed on the wall at their workstations. Two red, white, and blue revolving poles are mounted on the tops of the half wall. Other than that, the decor in the shop is sparse. At the back of the shop there's an eagle, globe, and anchor mounted to the wall on the side with the other barbers, Chris, Donald, and Ryan. A framed American flag that's folded into a triangle is mounted on the wall behind Mosiah and Bobby. It was given to him by the family of one of his friends who died during their tour in Iraq. A hand painted white wooden sign is hung across the back wall of the shop. It reads "Time is money." It is Mosiah's motto and a nod to the unspoken rule of the shop: Talk while you cut. If you can't talk and cut at the same time, then stop talking. Leo sits down in the empty chair and holds the broom between his knees.

He says, "If you want to know how much I make so bad, you can come go to work and find out for yourself."

"I got a job," Johnny says.

"No," Mosiah corrects him. "You have a job interview."

"Yeah, well, my moms knows the manager, so the interview is just a formality."

"If the interview was just a formality, you wouldn't be getting your hair cut," Mosiah says.

Johnny doesn't respond. He tilts his head the way Mosiah pulls him. His left leg shakes beneath the black cape.

"The only reason you want to work at Publix is because China and Dionna work there," Leo says. "I saw you talking to them at school."

"Oh, so it's about a girl," Mosiah says.

"No." Johnny moves his head away from Mosiah to glare at him and Leo.

"Boy, don't be snatching your head away from me. If you make me mess up your cut, you're not gon' like how low I have to take it to fix it. Don't nobody care about these lil' girls you out here chasin'. Every man in here has been there and done that."

"I know that's right," Chris, a barber across from Mosiah, cosigns.

"If you want to bag peoples groceries, push carts, and everything else, because you think it's gon' get you some, be my guest," Mosiah continues. "You'll learn once you get a taste that ain't no woman in the world, worth enough to lose money over."

"Hell yeah," Donald, a barber at the front of the shop, says. "You'll always lose money chasing women, but you'll never lose women chasing money."

"Didn't Chris Rock say that?" Johnny asks, looking up at Mosiah with his face screwed in disapproval.

"For all I know, Jesus could have said it," Donald answers. "Because that shit right there is gospel."

"Language," Mosiah says. "This is a family establishment."

"My bad, Boss," Donald says.

"Just look at Mo," Bobby, the barber behind Mosiah, says. "He been married to JoJo for what, six years, is it now, Mo?"

"Yeah," Mosiah answers. "Six years going on seven."

"Exactly," Bobby continues. "But truth be told, he woulda been married longer than that by now, had his old lady recognized his hustle when we were y'all age."

"What he mean, Boss?" Leo asks Mosiah.

"Bobby," Mosiah says, turning around to look at him, "You know you talk too damn much."

"But you know the talk I tell is the truth. Stop frontin' and school these young boys."

Mosiah rolls his eyes at Bobby. "You talk too damn much," he mutters under his breath. Mosiah shakes his head back and forth.

I am not the subject of conversation right now.

He turns the barber chair so Johnny is facing the wide glass mirror. He puts the shears down that he used to make the first dent in Johnny's long hair, and picks up his electric clippers.

Me and Jolene not even seeing eye to eye right now, and Bobby wanna put me on the spot. Today ain't the day for no fairytales and love stories. They can dead that.

Mosiah turns on the clippers and immediately goes to work, shearing away the rest of Johnny's hair until his natural curl pattern starts to pop, and there's only about two inches left. Mosiah squints his eyes and bites his bottom lip as he fades the back and the sides. He creates a gradient in Johnny's cut from the nape of his neck to the top of his hair, and then shuts the clippers off.

"So, Mo, you gon' tell us how you and Mrs. Jolene met, or nah?"

"I've been knowing Jolene since we were kids. We lived down the block from each other growing up, and went to the same schools our whole life."

"Yeah, but she wasn't checking for you until you came back from the Corps," Bobby says.

"Man, you want me to tell this story or do you want to?"

"You got it," Bobby says.

"And you got a client," Mosiah chastises, nodding his head toward the sign on the back wall.

He picks up his shears, once again, and clips away errant strands from Johnny's hair.

"So how come you and Mrs. Jolene didn't get together until after you got out of the military?" Leo asks.

Because she was being stupid.

"That's a question you need to ask my wife," Mosiah answers.

"But I'm asking you," Leo says.

Mosiah raises one eyebrow at Leo and looks around from him to the hair that covers the floor. Leo stands up from the chair and begins to sweep. Mosiah puts the hair shears back down on the countertop of his workstation and picks up his edgers.

"C'mon, Mo," Johnny says, looking at Mosiah through the mirror. "Tell us the story."

Got damnit, Bobby. These kids don't need to be in my business. They don't need to know Jolene didn't want me until Jemarcus stopped wanting her. I wasn't her first choice. I was safe. I was the right choice. The good guy.

"What you wanna know, man?" Mosiah sighs.

"What Bobby said. How come you and Mrs. Jolene didn't get together until after you came back home, if y'all knew each other forever."

"Jemarcus," Mosiah says flatly. "That's the guy JoJo got stuck on in middle school and high school."

"So how'd you get her back?" Johnny asks.

"He dumped her after she got pregnant, when we were in high school."

"You got with her when she was pregnant?" Johnny asks, looking up at Mosiah.

"Boy unscrew your face and turn around," Mosiah says. "You know you can't be moving while I'm doing your edge. You will walk out of here with a messed up head, and throw dirt on my name."

"My bad, Mo," Johnny says, turning back toward the mirror. "But what happened."

"Jemarcus dumped her, but we were still friends. I saw her in the hospital after she had the baby. I felt bad for her, but I was dating this girl named Cindy so everything was everything. She came back to school for senior year and graduated. She went to college and I went to the military. She came to my graduation from boot camp, and that surprised me. My mom told her about it, and after that we just kept in touch. I wrote her a few letters, but even when I didn't, no matter where I was in the world, she always managed to send me a letter, or a card, once a month. It was cool, because me and Cindy broke up before I left for boot camp. It was nice to get something from somebody else besides my mom and dad."

"Okay, but how did y'all finally get together?" Johnny asks.

"Damn, boy, you ask a lot of questions."

"Because you ain't saying nothing," Johnny says.

"Whatever man."

Mosiah turns off the edgers and places them back at his workstation. Mosiah picks up a jar of men's curling cream, opens it and scoops out a handful. He drops the dollop of cream into Johnny's hair, closes the jar, and then sets it back at his workstation.

"I didn't tell her when I came back home." Mosiah says working the product through Johnny's dry hair, until it soaks up the cream. "I was too messed up in the head after one of my guys, Nico, got killed."

"So, you had PTSD?" Leo asks, coming back to sit down in the empty chair in front of Mosiah.

"I don't know. Call it what you want. I came home and just didn't want to be bothered with nobody. I knew I wasn't going to re-enlist. And that school thing was never for me. I always cut my own hair, and did some other guys in the service, so I went to barber college. When I finished the program, I used all the money I saved in the service to open this place, and one day she walked in with TeeTee."

"She just walked in?" Donald asks. "You're sure it wasn't a setup?"

"Nah." Mosiah laughs, wiping his greasy hands on his smock.

He picks up his hair sponge and moves it in circles on Johnny's hair.

"I stopped writing her back after Nico. She didn't know I was home, and my folks knew better than to say anything to anybody. They gave me my space. So yeah, she just walked in with her son, trying to get his haircut, and we've been together ever since."

"So what does that have to do with me working at Publix?" Johnny asks.

"My man," Bobby says. "You not listening. Mo just said him and Jolene been together ever since the day she walked in this shop."

"Yeah. And?"

"And the name on the door says *Mo's Precision Cuts.* That means he owns it."

"So what," Johnny says.

"So what," Donald cuts in. "You think just any body can own a business?"

"Yeah," Johnny answers.

"Then if that's the case, then why you trying to work at Publix instead of being a young entrepreneur yourself."

"Because China and Dionna work there," Leo says.

"And that's exactly the point of this story," Ryan, the barber across from Bobby, says jumping into the conversation. He continues, "Mrs. Jolene saw Mo was a good guy, and had his own business when she couldn't even get her baby daddy to get his own son's hair cut. And they been together ever since."

"What business am I supposed to open at sixteen?" Johnny asks.

"Whatever you want to," Mosiah says. "The government don't care how old you are when you go into business. As long as they get they cut, they cool."

"Yeah. Well you weren't telling me to get my own business before. You were telling me to come work for you."

"I did, but that doesn't mean I want you to work for me forever."

"Seem like it, Leo still here," Johnny says.

"Because I wanna be," Leo says, sitting up straight in his chair.

"Calm down, y'all," Mosiah says.

He puts the sponge he'd been using to curl up the top of Johnny's hair down on the countertop and picks up his brush. He brushes the sides of Johnny's fade, powders his neck, and dusts off his collar, before pulling the cape from around him.

"Leo's still here because he's learning. He's an apprentice right now. Once he graduates Terry Parker, he can decide if he wants to go to barber college or do something else."

"Mo, you already know I'm going to barber school," Leo says. "This my chair right here."

Leo spins around in the chair.

"Either way," Mosiah continues. "He's learning the business and the craft at the same time. Anybody can open a barbershop. Not everybody can stay in business. If Leo wants to work in here after he finish school, he's got to build his own clientele just like every other man in here. They are independent contractors."

"But they still pay you," Johnny says.

"Booth rent," Mosiah says. "That goes to keeping the place up and running. And anytime they don't want to pay me and go out on their own, they can. That's why the chair Leo's sitting in is empty right now. The last guy had so many clients he was ready to go do his own thing. So he did, and it's all love."

"That's wassup," Johnny says. "But I'm still going to my interview tomorrow."

"He don't get it," Ryan says. "Mo, ain't no use in you even wasting your breath."

"Mo, some people are leaders and some people are followers," Leo says.

"Whatever," Johnny says. "I'm not cut out for service work. I don't want to sweep floors, cut hair, or clean buildings. I'm good."

"Boy, bagging groceries is service work," Mosiah says. "And I guarantee you'll be sweeping Publix and doing whatever else they decide they want you to do for minimum wage. But go on. You'll learn when China and Dionna don't want you, and you still working there."

"Man, Mo, why you gotta hate on me?" Johnny asks, standing up from the chair.

"It's not hate. You young, dumb, and full of . . . you know. I hope it works out for you," Mosiah says.

"Thanks, man," Johnny says.

Johnny hands Mosiah a twenty and a ten and walks to the door. The bell dings as he walks outside. Mosiah watches Johnny smooth the back of his bare neck. He watches until his black T-shirt, and dark denim shorts, disappear from the storefront.

"He'll figure it out one day," Leo says, standing up from his chair.

"You say that like you've lived two lives."

"Nah, it ain't that. It's just that I got common sense. Which means I know good sense when I hear it. Besides, China and Dionna got boyfriends anyway."

"They must be fine for you and Johnny to be checking for the same two girls," Mo says.

"Not as fine as the chicks I'm a get when I got my own spot like you."

"Keep dreaming, Leo. Keep dreaming."

"These ain't dreams, Mo. These are goals."

"What's the difference?" Mosiah asks.

"Dreams can last forever," Leo says. "Goals have a deadline."

"Look at you trying to sound deep," Bobby says behind Mosiah.

"Just make sure keeping my floor clean is one of your goals," Mosiah says.

"Spotless and shining. Always." Leo grins.

He walks to the back of the barbershop and grabs the broom from where he leaned it against the vending machine. Leo begins sweeping the floor, pushing the broom around the other barbers' stations. He sweeps the hair into a neat pile in the middle of the floor nearest Mosiah, then pulls the dust pan from his back pocket. Leo pushes all the hair, dust, dirt, candy wrappers, and other detritus dropped on the floor, intentionally or unintentionally, into the pan. He empties it into the trash can at Mosiah's station, and then shoves the pan back into his pocket. Sitting in the first chair at the front of the shop, Leo spins around with the broom between his knees and stops to face Mosiah.

He leans forward and asks, "So, Mo, why come you started your cleaning business if you were already doing good with the shop?"

"We had a kid," Mosiah answers.

"But you were still doing good with the shop, right?" Leo asks.

"Yeah."

"So why open a cleaning business?"

"Good is not the goal. Being comfortable and having my freedom is," Mosiah says.

Leo continues, "But of all the things you could have done, why not make the shop a franchise and open another one? Why cleaning?"

"For the exact same reason you're screwing your face up at me right now," Mosiah answers.

"And what's that?" Leo asks.

"Nobody likes to clean . . ."

"And you do?"

"I didn't say that. Nobody likes to clean, and people with money will pay somebody else to do it."

"I guess."

"There's nothing to guess. I own a barbershop and a commercial janitorial service. That's it. That's me."

"I still don't understand why."

"Because I like looking fresh and making money. Cutting hair keeps me fresh, and cleaning up after folks too lazy to do it themselves, keeps me paid."

"I get it."

"You don't have to. This is just my path. There's a lot of ways to make money in this world."

"I know that's right," Chris chimes in nodding his head.

"This is just the way I choose to make mine," Mosiah says. "It keeps the bills paid, a roof over my head, food on the table, and enough extra in my pocket that my lady's check is a non-factor."

"It always comes back down to the woman," Bobby says.

"I see," Leo says, with a smirk.

"Ha-ha. Y'all, got jokes," Mosiah says, dropping his brush in his container of barbicide. "I'm the only one in here who can say he's in a good relationship with no other complaints. My woman is happy, my kids are happy, and we live well."

Even if we're fighting right now.

"Yeah, okay," Leo says. "One day you'll have to break it down how you got Mrs. Jolene to stay down with you so long.

"Maybe one day I will," Mosiah says. "Maybe one day I will," he mutters to himself. Mosiah sits in his own chair and spins around toward the mirror. He looks over at the framed photo of himself, Jolene, Toussaint, and Lydia, taken when Lydia was first born. She was the star of the photo. Her two-week-old body was stretched across their hands. She was fast asleep and posed on their palms, with them all looking down at her. Mosiah looks from Lydia to Jolene in the picture. She was supposed to be looking completely down so that all that could be seen in the photo is the tops of their heads, the bridges of their noses, and the curve of their lips up into a smile, but Jolene cheated. In the photo he can still see her head lifted above him and Toussaint, her eyes on them, Toussaint especially, fearing he would drop their newborn baby; the sister he didn't want from the father he only half claimed.

Mosiah stares at Jolene's lifted eyes in the photo. The same deep, all knowing eyes she's had since they were in pre-school. She is his earliest memory. Her eyes, her face, her laugh, her smile. He doesn't remember being a baby. He has no recollection of his toddlerhood before Jolene; the girl who's cot was next to his. They used to have a staring contest as kids when they were supposed to be taking a nap. They would stare in each other's eyes, the loser was the one who fell asleep first. Jolene always lost. Mosiah remembers staring into her eyes until she closed them for good. He stared until her blinks got heavier, and lasted longer. He stared until he no longer saw the reflection of his own face in her pupils. He stared until he could see the moon and the stars and the depths of the ocean in the windows to her soul, until she shut him out and gave into sleep. It was only then that he allowed himself to be lulled away by the twinkling music of the instrumental lullabies playing in the nursery around them.

He loved her at three, the same way he loves her now at thirty. The only thing different about them is the time. She is still the same girl whose eyes he could get lost in forever. In the picture from Lydia's newborn photo shoot he sees love and a warning. "Please, don't drop my baby." It is the same look he saw when she first came into his shop with Toussaint and discovered he was home. There was love in her eyes, along with a plea from her heart. "Please don't hurt me or my baby."

7.

"Knock knock. Is anybody here?" Jolene asked aloud in the empty barbershop.

The sign glowing in the front door of the barbershop said open. She walked into the door that said *Mo's Precision Cuts* in the small strip mall on Fort Caroline Road with Toussaint sleeping on her shoulder. The bell connected to the door rang as she walked in, but the inside of the shop looked empty. Only one of the six workstations had any tools or products set up on the counter.

She shifted Toussaint's sleeping body from one shoulder to the other, and called out again, "Hello. Is anybody here? Are you open?"

"Yes, ma'am. We're open," Mosiah said, walking from the back room of the barbershop.

He dried his hands on a paper towel and shoved it into his back pocket.

"What do you need?" He asked looking up.

"Mosiah?" Jolene asked.

"Hey, JoJo," Mosiah said.

He watched the irritation etched in her face turn into shock and surprise, and then into a joyful smile. Her skin glowed as her teeth showed. Mosiah couldn't help from smiling himself.

"How long have you been back?" Jolene asked.

"Six months."

"You've been back six months and you didn't call and tell nobody, or even stop by the house?"

"I had a lot going on. I had to get myself together."

"Well, it seems like you're together now," Jolene said, looking around the empty barbershop.

From the smell inside, Jolene could tell the tile floor was freshly mopped and waxed from the way it shined. The entire shop had a smell of newness to it. The red chairs were still shiny, as if he'd just taken them out of the boxes and set them up. There were no worn wrinkles, cracks, tatters, or patches in the leather. The black futon in the waiting area where she stood didn't have any lint, or a noticeable sag from too many butts making a dent in the cushion. Her eyes directed her back to the bare walls and the lone workstation with the only set of clippers.

"How long have you been open?" She asked.

"Just signed the lease agreement last week for the space. I can't say I'm officially open yet because I don't have my license."

"So why would you get a space before you could actually cut hair."

"Because I wanted to have my space ready and waiting on me the day I finish the program. I can cover the rent here for six months. In the meantime, I've already advertised for barbers so they can work in here, and I can make money, until I can cut heads and make money myself."

"Sounds like you got it all figured out."

"Besides, the tax collector don't care if you licensed or not, if they getting their cut."

"What about inspections?"

"Right now, I'm not cutting hair."

"But your sign says you're open."

"I turned that on because I have a prospective barber coming in for an interview. Otherwise, the door is normally locked and the sign is off."

"Oh," Jolene said, shifting Toussaint to her other shoulder

"Is there something you need?" Mosiah asked.

"I came in because I saw the sign, and I need to get Toussaint's hair cut. But I guess you can't do it."

"It's after five. I don't think any inspectors are coming around now. If you want me to, I will," Mosiah said.

"Please," Jolene said.

"Come on back and have a seat in my chair. You're going to have to hold him. I don't have any booster seats for kids just yet."

"That's fine. He's asleep anyway. He wouldn't let me put him down even if you did."

Jolene followed Mosiah to his chair and sat down. She turned Toussaint around so that he sat in her lap with his sleeping head against her chest. He draped them with a black cape that said *Mo's Precision Cuts* across the front. The jagged handwriting font of the logo was scrawled beneath simple pictures of a comb, brush, hair shears, and clippers. The same emblem was stamped against the black smock Mosiah put on over his black T-shirt and jeans, and tied behind his waist.

"How low do you want it?" he asked.

"You can fade him down low so I don't have to worry about it next week, before graduation."

"Oh yeah?" Mosiah asked, grabbing his clippers and a guard from his workstation.

"Yeah," Jolene answered. "It took me an extra semester to finish. I was trying to do more at home and with Toussaint, so that it wasn't all on Granny Mae. Especially since she's watching Vaughn's baby now too."

"That's right. I forgot you told me your sister was pregnant?"

"Yeah, she had a little boy."

"What'd she name him?"

"Jovon."

"That's nice."

"Yeah."

"Hold his head steady for me," Mosiah said.

He turned on the clippers, and then stood beside Jolene to fade Toussaint's hair. He worked quickly so as not to wake the sleeping toddler, cutting the front of his hair first and then the back, before finishing with an edge. He stayed quiet as he worked. He breathed in her scent. Something floral still lingered, despite the late hour in the afternoon. He figured between classes indoors, and working indoors, she was never outside long enough to break a sweat; especially since it was only warm for a couple hours a day in December.

She still looks good though. I should have asked her for a picture while I was gone. It would have made those nights easier to go to sleep to looking at her eyes like when we were kids.

Mosiah finished Toussaint's haircut and brushed the left over fuzz down and around in the natural pattern of his head. He dusted them both off, before removing the cape from around their shoulders.

"All done," he said, shaking the hair from the cape onto the floor.

"How much do I owe you, Mo?" Jolene asked.

"Don't worry about it. I'm not supposed to be cutting anyway. This one's on the house."

"Thank you."

Jolene stood up and adjusted Toussaint in her arms. She pulled up the waistband of her jeans that had fallen down while she was sitting. Mosiah watched as she switched her thick hips from side to side, testing the elastic of the stretchy material to go back in place over her curves. He caught a glimpse of her pink thong, before she pulled her purple T-shirt back down over the exposed skin at her waist. Jolene adjusted Toussaint again, and picked up her purse from where she set it at his workstation.

Mosiah asked, "How old is lil' man, now?"

"Four," Jolene said.

"How come you getting him a haircut?"

"Because Jemarcus is unreliable."

"Mmhmm."

"Go ahead and say it." Jolene sighed.

"Say what?" Mosiah asked.

She watched him drape the cape over the back of his chair and walk to the back of the barbershop. He grabbed a broom and dust pan leaning against the wall, shoved the dust pan in his back pocket, and pushed the broom to where Jolene stood.

Still the same old Mo. Always nice, even when he doesn't have to be.

"You know you were the one who always warned me about Jemarcus. Even in eighth grade."

"That's because I was jealous," Mosiah said.

"I still should have listened," Jolene said.

"Too late now."

"I guess it is. Thanks for helping me out . . . with the haircut . . . for Toussaint I mean."

"Don't worry about it."

"Don't be a stranger, Mo." Jolene said as she walked toward the door.

Don't be a stranger.

Mosiah repeated her words to him as he watched her struggle to load the sleeping boy into his booster seat. By the time she had him strapped in and closed the back door, her clothes were all out of order again. He watched her jump her jeans back into position with the button at her navel, and the back waist sitting just below the top of her thong. She pulled up the front of her T-shirt that had fallen some to expose a lacy black bra. Mosiah watched from his stance in the middle of the barbershop, leaning on the broom, as Jolene pulled herself back together.

With her clothes in order, she turned to look at her reflection in the windows of her car. He watched as Jolene smoothed her hair around her face, opened the front passenger door, and threw her purse on the seat. She looked back at the barbershop and waved at Mosiah still standing in the middle of the floor with the broom.

Caught staring, Mosiah quickly bent down and pushed the hair from Toussaint's cut into the dust pan.

Don't be a stranger, he said replaying her words in his head. *Maybe I won't be. I been home too damn long anyway, to still be on this celibate bullshit.*

Mosiah stood up from the floor, and emptied the dust pan into the trash can at his station.

It ain't like Jemarcus in the picture no way. And if he is, he ain't doing his job. What man let's a woman take his son to get his haircut.

Mosiah shook his head and pushed the broom to the back of the barbershop and leaned it against the wall. He hung the dust pan on the hook of a mounted coat rack, and then walked to his station. He adjusted his pants and underwear from the tightening knot that began at his groin as he watched Jolene leave.

Don't be a stranger.

Her words played a refrain in his head as he went to work organizing his space, and cleaning his brush and his clippers. He was so focused on the task in his hands and her voice in his head he didn't hear the bell ring as the door to barbershop was opened a second time.

"Hey, I'm here about the job for barbers."

Mosiah turned around. "Bobby, man. What the hell you doing here?"

"Trying to work," Bobby said. "How long you been back?"

"Six months."

Mosiah walked up to Bobby, slapped his hand, and clapped his back for a hug. Bobby was his best friend from high school, the one he played football with for all four years. They both held down the O-line. Bobby dreamed of playing in college at Alabama, but an injury senior year and piss-poor grades left him stuck in Jacksonville, going to community college, and playing pick-up games through a community league, based out of whichever park district was nearest to his neighborhood.

Bobby said, "Your black ass been back six months and you don't call nobody. People wondering how you doing and everything. We don't know if you dead or alive. You know it's a war going on."

"No shit," Mosiah said. "What you got there? Man, is that a résumé?"

"Yeah. I had to come correct. I didn't know this was your spot."

"So you would've come some other way if you knew I was the employer beforehand?"

"Nah, man. It ain't even like that," Bobby said. He wiped his brow of the imaginary sweat that wasn't beading anywhere on his skin

"Chill out, man," Mosiah said. "I'm just fucking with you."

"You got me nervous and shit," Bobby said, wiping his palms on his slacks.

"I see. You almost got a suit on."

"I try to clean up proper when I'm about business."

"You looking good, man."

Mosiah nodded his head in approval of Bobby's black slacks, and long sleeved white button-down shirt. The shirt was starched and pressed, and buttoned to the top, despite Bobby's thick neck hanging over the collar. His hair was cut short, and his full beard was combed out and trimmed to perfection. Mosiah looked at his rounded face and genial smile, and saw the same friend he played side by side with under the Friday night lights. Always joking, always eager, always supportive.

"When you finish the program?" Bobby asked.

"I haven't yet. I'm just holding my spot until I get my license, so I don't have to work for nobody else once I do."

"Man, you always was a scheming, planning, plotting, motherfucker," Bobby said, sitting down in one of the barber chairs.

"Ain't no scheme. If you fail to plan, then you plan to fail, and I ain't about failing shit. Uncle Sam got his four years outta me. That's all he getting too."

"I heard that."

"So, why you wanna work for me?" Mosiah asked.

"Oh, is this the interview part now?" Bobby asked with a smirk.

"Hell yeah," Mosiah said.

"Hol' up. Wait a minute then. Before we start. Who was shawty that walked out when I was pulling up?"

"Oh, you saw her?"

"Every man on this side of the Atlantic saw all that ass in them jeans."

"Man, you know who that is," Mosiah said.

"Who?" Bobby asked.

"JoJo," Mosiah said.

"Who the fuck is Jo . . . Oh snap. You mean Jolene."

"The one and only."

"Oh, so y'all together now?"

"Not yet," Mosiah answered.

"What you mean, not yet?"

"Just what the fuck I said. Not yet. I hadn't even told her I was back. She just walked in on a whim."

"Naw, man, that ain't no whim. That's what girls be calling that kismet shit."

"Call it what you want. I know I'm calling her."

"Don't she got a shorty though?"

"Yeah. He's four."

"You might wanna slow your roll then," Bobby said. "You don't wanna be caught up in no baby daddy shit."

"Don't seem like Jemarcus in the picture. And even if he is, I can handle it."

"Then get it how you live then. Get it how you live."

"Oh, I will. She already told me don't be a stranger. She ain't got to tell me twice, and I already know where she stay."

"Seems like you got a nice little situation getting ready pop off."

"Nah. Ain't no situation. That's about to be my wife," Mosiah said, with a certainty that surprised himself

What did I just say? My wife? I haven't even been on a date in four years.

"Man, you tripping. You been gone too long talking about that's your wife. How about you run through some hos for awhile, before you get to committing to one chick and what not. Especially a chick with a kid."

"Ain't no need, man. I already know what I want. I think I've known since I was three. Was just waiting on her to be ready."

"That's some *Lifetime* movie type love shit," Bobby said. "That, or the war really fucked you up."

"Nah. Death just has a way of putting life in perspective."

"Who died?" Bobby asked.

"Don't worry about it. You ready to do this interview, or what?"

"No doubt."

"Good. Wait right up there in the waiting area so I can finish putting my stuff away, and then we'll get to it."

"Bet."

Bobby walked to the front of the shop as Mosiah turned around to finish cleaning up his workstation, his mind racing over his words.

My wife. I didn't see that coming. Maybe I did. But I for damn sure didn't mean to tell Bobby. Whatever. It's out in the universe now.

Mosiah placed his clippers and edgers back into the holes cut into the countertops for his tools, and dusted his fingers across the countertop. His words and her words played on repeat in his mind as he untied his smock and draped it across the back of his chair.

Don't be a stranger.

That's about to be my wife.

Mosiah sighed deeply, then walked to the front of the shop where Bobby waited for him. His heart and his mind were disconnected from the interview; interrupted by the kismet connection of the woman who left.

8.

"Let's clean the glass stuff first and then the floors. In the bathrooms and the offices," Mosiah directs. "We can empty the trash cans as we go."

"No problem, Boss," Ricky says.

Mosiah watches as he disappears with Michael toward the bathrooms of the building they're cleaning. Sterling Broadcast Communications is the parent company of the news station Mosiah recently won the cleaning contract for. It is their first night on the job. Typically, they clean commercial office buildings where the workers leave by five, and he and his crew are left alone to do their jobs. A convenient condition that allows them to leave usually within an hour of arriving. This is the first time he's been in an office building where employees were still around, and actively working when he and his crew arrived.

Mosiah watches as Ricky pushes the rolling yellow mop bucket, and Michael pushes the large garbage can out of the main space of the newsroom, toward a hallway where the cubicles of the nine to five workers have long been vacated. Both wear utility belts packed with rubber gloves, paper towels, dust mitts, and brandless bottles of all-purpose cleaner. Anthony and Justin move toward the conference rooms and private offices, pushing a garbage can and a vacuum cleaner. The five of them together make up the "The Walker Way Cleaning Service." Mosiah remains in the middle of the large warehouse style building, and begins to dust and clean the pods of cubicles meant to engender a sense of community, while also maintaining each workers' individual space and identity.

"Good evening," he says to a man and woman sitting in two of the pod spaces toward the back of the room.

"Hey," the man says. "You guys are new."

"We are," Mosiah says. "Today is our first day."

"Welcome," the man says, extending his hand. "I'm Linden."

"Nice to meet you," Mosiah says, shaking his hand.

"I'm Tarren," the woman says, extending her hand.

"Mosiah."

"That's a different name," Tarren says.

"It means savior, or gift of God."

"Hmm," Tarren says. "That's religious."

"What can I say?" Mosiah shrugs. "We live in the South and my dad's a preacher. Nice meeting y'all."

"You too," Linden says.

Mosiah pushes his garbage can and vacuum cleaner to the empty set of pods across from Tarren and Linden. He puts the wireless headphones he had around his neck over his ears, and pulls his phone out of the front pocket of his jumpsuit. He scrolls through his music until he finds an album that matches his mood. He skips the first track of the critically acclaimed rap album and chooses track two, with a bass heavy melody, and a sample from the sixties; a Nina Simone song with her lyrics chopped and screwed. Mosiah cranks the music in his ear and lets the mood and message of the song overtake him as he works. His hands dust and wipe, spray and clean, polish and shine, as the music takes him back to the barbershop.

Why open a cleaning business?

The question was from the honest mouth, and the earnest eyes of his eager apprentice, trying to learn his own version of a zero sum game for ten dollars an hour. It is a question Mosiah has become comfortable with being asked, over and over, by various people. Jolene asked him. Her parents asked him. His parents asked him. Toussaint asked him. Even Jemarcus asked him with a smirk across his face, and bouncing eyes that belied how little he thought of the man who chose to raise his own son. He saw disgust in the eyes of those who only thought of him as a janitor, rather than an entrepreneur.

If I were them, I would look down on me too.

"Financial freedom, my only hope. Fuck living rich and dying broke."

Mosiah mumbles his favorite part of the song as he moves over to the section of pods where Tarren and Linden sit. He works quickly around them, bopping his head to the music, ignoring the TV's on every desk, the same channel playing on each one. Mosiah shoves his dust mitt and cleaner into the slots on his utility belt, empties the trash can beneath Tarren's desk, and then cuts on his vacuum cleaner. He glances briefly at the TV and sees a woman who reminds him of a skinny version of Jolene. The way she used to look in high school, except the woman on the TV is wearing a bad wig with too many blonde and brown highlights for her honeyed skin. Jolene always kept her hair it's natural off black color. He loved it when she was pregnant, and her long hair draped her fattening face and spreading nose.

It was in the hospital, after she delivered Lydia, that he got the idea for the cleaning business. His father, Reverend Paul Alan Walker, came to visit him alone, without his mother. Mosiah remembers Jolene had just fallen asleep with Lydia still in her arms when his dad walked into the room, unaccompanied.

"Where's Mom?" Mosiah asked.

"At home, I suppose," his dad answered. "She doesn't know I'm here."

"I bet she doesn't," Mosiah said. "You know she'd kill you coming up here to see her grand-baby without her."

"I know," his dad said.

Mosiah took Lydia from Jolene and held her in his arms as he sat on the couch with his father. It was then, after all the small talk that could be made was done, that his father revealed the true reason for his solo visit.

"You're a daddy now," Reverend Walker said.

"I've been a daddy," Mosiah answered.

"Yeah, but Toussaint isn't really yours. You adopted him and gave him our name, but it's not the same as when you hold your own seed."

Mosiah nodded as his father started his lecture the same way he started his sermons: with an observation leading to a larger idea and point.

Reverend Walker continued, "This little girl here means you have new responsibilities. You have new priorities, and that's going to be a problem."

"What do you mean?" Mosiah asked.

"You're a daddy to Toussaint because you had to be to get Jolene. I get it. You've loved her since before you knew what the word love meant. So to love her, you had to love him. They were a package deal. Loving one means you had to love the other. But with Lydia, it's a whole new ball game. You don't think you love her more than Toussaint, but you do. You don't think that you will treat her differently, but you will. You don't think that you will be harder on him, and more lenient on her, because she's your blood and he's not, but it will happen."

"Daddy, you sound like you got a whole 'nother family Mama and I don't know about."

"No. I've just got a flock of families that have failed because they didn't know how to blend and love everybody equally, or as close to it as possible."

"So how do I not be that way?" Mosiah asked.

"You have to recognize that's our human flaw to care for our own more than somebody else's forgotten leftovers, and work twice as hard to love that one twice as much, so they don't ever feel left out, or unloved."

"I already work my ass off at the shop."

"But is it enough. Is it enough for you, Jolene, Toussaint, and now Lydia?"

Mosiah didn't answer then, but the seed was planted. In the hospital room, after his father left, he began thinking of other things to do, other businesses to start, other avenues of income to make up what would become his apparently inherent biases toward his children. The child he made, and the child he chose to raise. It wasn't until he saw the hospital cleaning crew mopping the halls that he knew he'd found what he needed to do. He couldn't tell Leo and Johnny that he wanted to clean because that wasn't true. The cleaning business was his calling to make sure Lydia never questioned his capacity to provide all she dreamed, that Toussaint never questioned his loyalty or his love to him, and that Jolene never questioned his love for her and the family she settled to make for the man she decided to love.

Jolene, the girl, the woman his father knew he loved before he could even understand the sobering gravity of what the word love even meant. With the same fire he had to will himself to stay awake on his daycare cot, so that he could watch her fall asleep first, is the same fire he gave to his anger when she chose Jemarcus over him in the eighth grade. He found that same fire again and gave it back to his heart to rekindle the eternal flame he carried for her as he traipsed across the world, fighting another man's war, sustaining himself on her words, though he told himself she was just being nice.

"Do I find it so hard," Mosiah sings to himself as the chilling title track of the album begins to play in his headphones.

The wailing songstress of the flipped UK soul band drowns out the sound of Mosiah's vacuum as he moves away from the pods, and toward the center piece in the room. The raised platform of an octagon with computer-lined desks, making up the perimeter of the shape. Mosiah vacuums around the octagon and then steps up on the platform to vacuum the center of it, before dusting the desks on the periphery. From here he can see Anthony and Justin working their way down toward the studio where Jolene's skinny doppelgänger is at work on set. Three TV's are suspended from the ceiling above him. One on the channel showing the woman at work just a few feet away from him, another a split of screens on the broadcast networks of the apparent competition, showing primetime sit-coms or dramas, and the third shows cable news commentators in another screen split. The only sound Mosiah hears is from his headphones; rap and wailing. He told his crews from day one "Do what you need to do to get the job done, so we can all go home." Justin and Anthony both sport headphones, one of them listening to a podcast, and another to heavy metal.

Ricky and Michael turn the bend back into the newsroom. Mosiah takes one of his headphones down.

He says, "You two, take the elevator and do upstairs. Anthony and Justin, if you're done with those offices, go with them."

"We're going," Anthony says.

"I'll finish up down here, with that big room and the studio. We should be out of here in about half an hour."

"Right on," Ricky says.

Mosiah puts his headphones back on as the sample of a song he grew up hearing played on Sunday mornings, comes through his ears. Mosiah works his way to the large empty area behind the news studio. He vacuums in wide arcing strokes, until the room is left smelling like the lavender scented powder he coated the floor with to make sure he didn't miss any spots. Mosiah cuts the vacuum off and leaves his garbage can in the middle of the empty room, and walks to the studio. He waits on the edge, away from the anchor at the desk, out of view of the cameras until the show goes off. He looks at the clock face of his smart watch. It reads 8:57.

I should be home before ten. I may need to hire another crew to do this job. By the time I get home, everybody is going to be asleep. But me and Jolene need to talk. I don't know why that woman is so damn hardheaded. She never listens, even when it's for her own damn good. It's not like I said something was wrong. For all we know, it could just be a pimple. But it doesn't hurt to go get it checked out. Instead of making a damn appointment like she said she would, she goes to see her therapist. The old lady from her church. Who knows what she's telling my wife.

Mosiah feels a tap on his arm. He looks down to see the anchor woman who was at the desk, standing in front of him. He pulls his phone out of his pocket and turns the music off.

"Hello," she says, once he takes down his headphones. "I'm Naomi."

"I know," Mosiah says.

"And you are?" Naomi asks.

"Mosiah," he says, steeling himself to her constant pets and pats.

"Nice to meet you. Do you need anything?"

"Nope. I was waiting for you to finish your show so I can clean the studio, and go home to my family."

"Oh, you have kids?" Naomi asks. "How many?"

"My wife and I have a boy and a girl."

"Good for you," Naomi says, pulling her hand away from his shoulders.

"Yeah," Mosiah says with a smirk. "You have a good night."

Naomi walks away from Mosiah, stomping her bare feet across the thin peasy carpet with her heels in her hand.

She looks better on TV than she does in person. Taller too. All that damn makeup. She'd probably look better without it. Jo for damn sure don't need it.

Mosiah places his headphones on his ears and pulls the phone out of his pocket. He scrolls the albums on his music app until he finds what he's looking for. The second album of a nearly forgotten 2000's neo-soul crooner. Once again, his aural senses are assaulted, this time by an acoustic guitar, accompanied by simple piano keys and harmonious melodies, the music of his musing. Mosiah quickly sprays and wipes down the glass anchor desk, the high-top rolling chairs, and the white leather couches of a little used section of the set off to the side, away from the main desk. The entire time, the whining sentiments of a half crazy man who turned a friend into a lover, play on repeat.

"You used to laugh/now you get mad/Damn/I just want my friend back," Mosiah sings to himself as he works.

The tenor his mother honed as the choir director in his father's church, he puts to use to comfort himself. Mosiah works, singing the song that got him over the high school heartbreak, that his one time best friend was pregnant by a boy who didn't deserve her. The song he sang to himself when he was on desert battlefields waiting to get her letter. The song he played relentlessly when she found him by accident and stoked the flames of their relationship that never was. The song he plays now, that she won't listen to him, won't confide in him, and won't take his advice, when all he wants for her is the best.

"We used to chill/and be down for whatever/ whenever/together/yeah."

Why is she so fucking difficult? I just wish she'd go figure out what's wrong. If it's nothing, we can move on. I swear, I hate this uncertain shit. I should have just stayed in the military. Reenlisted like everyone else in my platoon. I'd have my orders, and my black and white life back. Do something good, get promoted. Fuck up, pay the consequences. This gray area real world shit is for the birds.

"Boss, you good?" Ricky asks, lifting one of the ears of Mosiah's headphones.

"Whoa, man. Damn!" Mosiah says, jumping. "You know better than to sneak up on me like that."

"My bad. I thought something was wrong. Sound like you crying in here."

"Whatever, man, you know I sound good. You just jealous with your no talent having ass."

"Yeah, man, whatever," Ricky says. "We finished upstairs."

"Good. I'm done in here. Let's put the stuff away, bag up this trash, and get it to the dumpster so we can go."

"Cool," Ricky says.

This is definitely too long of a day for me. I need to put an ad out for another man ASAP.

Mosiah lifts his headphones as the song he put on repeat automatically starts over again. He pushes his trash can behind his two crews to the janitorial closet, where they will keep their supplies as long as they have the contract. Five bags of garbage sit at their feet after they close the closet. Each man grabs a bag and heads toward the front door. Mosiah takes one ear down from his headphones and waves his hand at the people sitting in the sparsely populated newsroom.

"Y'all, have a good night," he says.

A chorus of "you too's" follows as he walks out behind Ricky, Michael, Anthony, and Justin.

"Have a good night, Mosiah," says a lone female voice.

Mosiah raises his hand in the air again and waves behind him, without turning around to acknowledge Naomi directly. He smiles to himself and shakes his head.

Lady, I got too many problems as it is to entertain you.

Mosiah puts his headphones back on and hums along with the melancholy melody of his favorite sad song, emboldened to not end up like the protagonist in the chorus.

We're going to figure this out one way or another.

9.

"Jo, what's wrong?" Mosiah asks coming through the front door.

"Nothing, I was waiting on you," Jolene says, sitting up on an elbow.

"You didn't have to do that," Mosiah says, closing the door behind him. "I told you I would be coming in late because of the new contract we picked up."

"I know. Where was it again?"

"The news station. The one that got the new black woman everybody's been talking about."

"Oh yeah," Jolene says.

Mosiah kicks off his work boots at the front door and walks over to sit by Jolene. She lifts her head from the beige sofa and makes room for him to sit down, then lays her head in his lap.

"Yeah. She kind of looks like you. But when I saw her up close, I realized it was more makeup than anything else."

"She's too skinny to look like me," Jolene says.

"Wait until she has some babies," Mosiah says. "I'm sure she'll round out just like you did."

"Is she married?"

"Not at all," Mosiah says, exaggerating the last word.

"Why'd you say it like that?"

"I guess she called herself trying to take your husband."

"You got hit on today?" Jolene asks, sitting all the way up. "Ooh. Ow," she says, gripping her side.

"What's wrong?" Mosiah asks.

"Nothing. Just a sharp pain."

"How long has that been going on?"

"It just started tonight."

"On the side that you're holding?"

Jolene winces. "Yes," she says, then lets out a deep guttural sigh.

"And yet you still haven't called the doctor."

Mosiah sighs and huffs to himself. *This has gone on long enough.* He stands up from the couch and walks behind Jolene to the kitchen. He opens the refrigerator door and pulls out a green bottle of beer. Popping the top with his hand, he takes a long smooth swig.

"Is that your answer to everything?" Jolene asks, not turning around to look behind her. "Call the doctor."

"It will be every time you complain about something, without getting that thing checked out."

"Mo, it's nothing. It's almost gone."

"But it's not," Mosiah says.

You probably haven't even checked, he thinks to himself. *You only do things when they're absolutely necessary, and even then, you make it a chore.*

Mosiah watches Jolene from where he stands, leaning against the refrigerator. Her earth toned, striped scarf is tied securely on her head, protecting her strands, edges, and flyaways from the elements that make up the damaging fibers of the couch cushions or her pillow case, for when she finally gets in the bed. The sleeveless straps of her terry cloth baby doll night-gown reveal slightly hunched shoulders. From his favorite vantage point, when he stands behind her, he can tell if she's relaxed, when he has a clear view of her collarbone. Right now, that view is obstructed by her raised shoulders toward her ears. It is his signal that he should tread lightly into the uncertain waters of the subject matter they're wading into. He can see in her physical form that she will strike back against his predatory posture, that is ready to strike to save the best part of himself: her.

Mosiah drains the beer bottle, opens the refrigerator and grabs a second. After popping the top and taking a swig, he comes back to the living room, back to his wife, back to the couch that will serve as their battleground.

"Why won't you call the doctor to make an appointment?" he asks.

"Because I just had my annual exam two months ago. The doctor did my pap and breast exam then, and didn't even say anything to me about something being off or abnormal."

"What's that supposed to mean?"

"It means . . . if a medical professional didn't find anything wrong with me, I doubt you have."

He sees the pride etched in the smirk on her face that says "check mate, Mo." He doesn't back down.

"A lot can change in two months," Mosiah says. "Wouldn't you rather know for sure that nothing is wrong, instead of having all of these strange symptoms for something you can't call is the matter."

"Ignorance is bliss," Jolene says.

"And firemen burn books in the future," Mosiah retorts.

Jolene sighs. "What's your point?"

"My point is . . . there is a reason you're afraid to pick up the phone and call for an appointment over something the size of a large nose pimple."

"I'm not afraid," Jolene says, "I'm just busy; and when I'm not busy, I'm tired."

"Jolene, I just worked damn near fourteen hours. You don't think I'm tired? I am. But I still have the time to make sure I eat, I feel well, and to make sure you've done the same."

"I'm not, not acknowledging that you've just worked fourteen hours. But let's not forget I'm up before you; I'm out of the door before you. I have a much more strenuous and stressful job than you do, and when that's over I have Toussaint and Lydia. A job that will never end, no matter how big or how old they get."

"Jolene! This is not about who works longer or harder hours at their jobs; inside or outside of this house."

Because it's me, Mosiah thinks continuing the conversation with himself. *I'm the one with two businesses, busting my ass to keep everybody else around here happy.*

He says, "This is about why you won't go see a damn doctor, when you have insurance for everything else you want to use it for."

Jolene knows Mosiah is referring to Doctor Fisher. She doesn't shake her head, hunch her shoulders, or let any activity in her body show how much she resents his jab at her chosen form of healing. He's known her long enough, and knows why she's opposed to other, more traditional procedures steeped in medical dogma that still leave patients without answers. And if he's forgotten, all it takes is one look at her unnecessary C-section scar between the lines of her stretch marks for him to be reminded why some doctors are not for everyone. She sighs her unspoken thoughts into the closed lips of her mouth.

What I do to maintain my sanity and my peace is my business. Some people drink. Some people eat. Some people exercise. Some people go to therapy. And some people do it all.

Mosiah places the half-empty bottle of beer beside his feet on the dark mahogany hardwood floors. He unzips the top of his work suit and pulls his arms out. Beer back in his hand, he reclines on the sofa with his chest, arms, and back exposed. He closes his eyes and takes another sip, and another sip, then drains the bottle.

He says, "Tell me what's so hard about picking up the phone, calling the doctor, and making an appointment. What is so stressful or strenuous about that? How long does it take to dial seven numbers and say "see me?""

"I never said it was hard," Jolene rebuts. "I said I don't have time for it. I get up, get dressed, go to work, and teach all day. After my classes are over at school, I take the little thirty minutes I have before I have to get Toussaint and Lydia to respond to the people on blackboard for my masters. I leave work, I go get them, and then usually I have to go by and help Mama and Daddy with Granny Mae, because Vaughn and Tanya rarely do. Some nights I have choir rehearsal, some days Toussaint has football practice, and even if we ever can come straight home, they need to eat, the house needs to be cleaned, clothes washed, and they gotta get to bed. It's not until all of that is over that I can even work on whatever assignment or paper we have for the week, so I can turn it in on time. And then I still have to grade my own students' work, so you tell me where in all that time, I'm supposed to remember to make an appointment for something that's not even bothering me."

"You made an appointment for your annual exam two months ago, didn't you? You always manage to get Lydia to all of her well-child checks, and Toussaint to whatever sports physical or whatever else he needs, don't you? So if you can make their appointments and yours, then why are you too busy to make another one now."

"I just told you why."

"You should never be too busy to take care of yourself."

"How can I take care of me when I have to take care of everybody in this house, including you?"

"So, I'm not working to take care of everybody in the house too? Including you? You can't even fix your mouth to say those words, because you know they're not true."

"I never said anything like that. I don't discount what you do. All I'm saying is don't discount everything I've got going on."

"I'm not, Jo. But it's one phone call. And one appointment. Surely, you have time enough for that."

"If I remember to do it, I'll call. If it's such a big deal to you, why don't you make the damn appointment and just let me know when to show up."

"You ain't said nothing but a word," Mosiah says, standing up. "I'm going to bed."

Jolene swings her feet back on the sofa in the space he vacated and lays back down.

"You coming?" Mosiah asks.

"In a little bit."

She listens to his feet pad up the stairs and walk to their room. The wooden floorboards, beneath the carpet on the second floor, creak from the houses age, and potentially poor construction.

I don't know why he keeps making a big deal out of nothing. If it was something serious. I would know. It's my damn body.

I would know.

I would know if something was wrong before anybody else. I just need to rest.

Jolene justifies her pain, her dizziness, and her shortness of breath to a lack of rest and sleep. She closes her eyes as the sounds of the shower come on above her head. Sighing deeply, she allows the consonant dissonance she's created convince her that she has won the battle and in turn the war over her body and her health, and what is the best for herself.

I need Doctor Fisher a whole helluva lot more than I need to be laid up on somebody's exam table, them poking at me, trying to pop a pimple I can drain with a needle.

In the shower, Mosiah washes away the dirt and the dust of the day down the drain. He stands beneath the rain showerhead and lets the gentle drops of water fall down his entire body. It soaks his head and face, washing the grease he uses in his hair to keep his scalp soothed, and his hair laid, into his eyes. The product stings as it pollutes his pupils. Mosiah resists the urge to wipe his face and lets the water do its work, and eventually rinse away the pain.

There's got to be more to it than just stubbornness. This is one of the dumbest arguments we've ever had. I just want to know she's okay. That it's nothing serious.

Fuck it.

If she don't care. I don't care. We can just get back to being us.

But I can't pretend like this is not an issue. Like I'm not going to think about it. Like I'm not going to feel it when I touch her. Hell, I'll probably be looking for it. When you know something, you can't unknow it.

Mosiah turns the cooling water off and gets out of the shower. He tracks his wet body through the bathroom and back into the bedroom, not bothering to dry off. He grabs underwear from the chest of drawers, pulls them on, and gets in the bed. He closes his eyes but sleep eludes him. The sleep he craves to put a period on the day, plays keep away. His mind races with the best and the worst of what could happen to Jolene.

We can't just ignore it, because I can't just ignore it.

I'll give her until noon. If she hasn't called, I will.

He hums to himself. An uptempo R&B song from a movie comes to his mind. He hums the verse until he gets to the chorus. The only part of the song where he knows the words.

"Wherever you run/that's where I'll go."

Mosiah sings and hums until his yawns outnumber his words and sleep finally subsumes him.

This is how Jolene finds Mosiah when she finally comes into the room. Sleeping on his side. His body facing where her body should be. She creeps across the room to the bed. In the darkness, she feels her way for the handle of the nightstand and pulls it open. Jolene grabs her journal, with the pen inside, closes the drawer and creeps back out of the room. She takes the stairs to the first floor, to the kitchen, where a cup of freshly brewed tea leaves are steeping for her in a mug. The only light on in the house is the lamp above the range, and the glow of the time from both the stove and microwave. Two-thirty a.m. flashes at her in blue-green numbers as she sits at the head of the table, still tired, though she is fully awake.

May 9,

It's 2:30 in the damn morning and I'm wide awake, while he's sleeping like a baby. Isn't that always how it goes? Men start an argument and pick fights, and then go to sleep like nothing even happened. Now here I am still up, trying to figure out what happened, what went wrong, what did I do now? What didn't I do that I should have done, and he's just sleep.

Maybe I should call the doctor. That would make him happy and prove to him that nothing's wrong. I just need to lose some weight, drink more water, and stop eating junk my body feels the need to purge in the most awkward of ways.

But what if something is wrong?

I felt it before he did. And it hasn't gone away.

Maybe I should call Doctor VanBuren again, and tell him to check it out. It couldn't hurt. But I know I'm going to be pissed if it's nothing, like I said, and I wasted my time. I don't have time to waste. Between the kids, my school, going to school, church and Granny Mae, I don't have spare moments. I barely had time to see Doctor Fisher with all I've got going on. Hell, I didn't even stay for that whole appointment.

Everybody just wants too much of me. I don't mind giving, but damn if I'm not empty. And people keep taking what I don't even have left. Especially Mo. That's what he was designed to do. Take. Just like Jemarcus. And Daddy. I used to hear Mama up late at night, early in the morning. She said she was praying, but she was always crying, probably because Daddy kept taking, even what was not his.

She only let it slip once when she caught me crying over Jemarcus, after he missed something with me and Toussaint. I don't even remember.

I was at the little table in the kitchen crying, rocking Toussaint to sleep in my arms when she walked in. I tried to wipe my face, but she already saw me. She just sat down at the table and let me get it out.

Then she said, "Jolene, men are takers by nature. While women are givers."

All I could say to her then with my pitiful ass, teary eyes was, "He's taken everything I've got, and I've got nothing left to give."

She said, "Women by design are meant to receive, but the other side of that reception is giving. We give, and we give, and we give, and we give, and they take, and they take, and they take, and they take. They take the very essence from your body, and stuff it in their drawls. They take pieces of your soul and zip it in their jeans, like you're just another zipless fuck that didn't mean much."

It was one of the few times I'd heard Mama curse, but she just kept on like she didn't even say nothing.

She said, "Stop giving what you don't have, and receiving what's not meant for you."

After that, she just got up from the table and walked away like nothing ever happened. Like she didn't even say anything.

I thought that just applied to Jemarucs, but maybe it applies to Mo too. He's a man. He takes.

But he's given too. More than I could have ever imagined. More than I could have ever dreamed. And all he wants is for me to take care of myself.

That's not too much to ask. Is it?

The question is, what will he ask for next, and will I have it to give? There's always something else. Another request. Even if this one is for me, the next one may not be.

But that's marriage. Right? Give and take. We both have to take as much as we give. That's the only way this will work. It's the only way it's been working. The only way it should work.

10.

Jolene's two word response to his text message confirms what Mosiah already knew he would have to do. He sits in his small office at the back of the barbershop, across from the bathroom. The room was once a storage closet before he repurposed it into his office. Mosiah reclines in his leather desk chair, his head is stretched back on the built-in pillow cushion, and his feet are extended in front of him. His work smock is still tied around his neck and waist as he rests away from the men and their clients in the shop.

Papers are stacked in neat piles behind the laptop on the desk made of reclaimed wood. There is the pile of papers for him to keep track of his clients, a small black appointment book he rarely uses now that he's created a website with a portal for clients to book online, and then the pile of bills for the shop. Off to the side is a pile of manila folders with the information of each barber, and finally, there is a pile of résumés for applicants looking to replace the barber who left to open his own shop. That pile he's been waiting to go through, waiting to see if Leo is serious about going to barber college after high school. If Leo does go to barber college, Mosiah will throw the pile of résumés in the trash, if he does not, he will begin to schedule interviews for someone to take the first chair in front of him. He knows he's bringing in enough cash to hold off the three weeks until Leo's graduation, and a year if Leo is serious about working for him.

It's all on you, Leo.

Mosiah sits up in his chair and scribbles his finger against the mouse pad built into his laptop, to bring the screen to life. He opens an internet browser and searches for hospitals, until he finds the number of the one he wants.

Am I really going to do this or should I give her more time?

She's been stalling for a week . . . Maybe more.

Just call and see what they say. If it's not meant to be, they won't let you make the appointment.

Mosiah enters the ten digits on his phone. He hesitates. His finger hovers over the green send button, suspended in the air, tentative. It is as if his finger has become his brain, contemplating all possible scenarios before finally pressing dial. His heart rate increases with the first ring of the phone. It rings a second time, and nearly a third before a pleasant voice; young, southernly sweet, and overly mannered takes over.

"Good Morning, Mayo Clinic, how may I direct your call?"

"Umm . . ." Mosiah stumbles. He coughs.

"How may I direct your call?"

Mosiah coughs once, and then twice before clearing his throat. "Umm . . . Do you allow spouses to make appointment for patients?"

"Why sure, let me get you over to the central appointment line."

The line clicks and classical piano music takes over before the ringing starts again. His heart races. Another voice comes over the line, rough with age and gravelly from cigar smoke and alcohol.

"Mayo Clinic, how may I help you."

Mosiah coughs. He works to clear his unchecked anxiety so that his voice comes out in a normal authoritative tone.

"Hello." He hears in his ear.

He opens his mouth, but all that comes out is another forced cough. It's forced from the back of his throat, where his fear rises and his courage diminishes with each passing second, marked by the breath on the other end of the phone, waiting for him to speak. Mosiah coughs. "Sorry," he strains. "I'm uh . . . Umm . . . I'm calling to make an appointment."

"Sir, is it for you?"

"No," Mosiah answers. "It's for my wife."

"Is she a current patient here?"

"No."

"Okay, we can schedule her for you if you like."

"Yes, please," Mosiah answers.

"What is her concern?"

It's not her concern, it's mine.

Mosiah answers, "Well, we found a bump. About the size of a large pimple. She didn't know what it was and so we want to get it checked out. To be sure."

"You would like to schedule a mammogram for your wife?"

"If I can, please," Mosiah says.

"Yes, sir. We'll just need some information from you first."

Mosiah sighs, still trying to clear his neurotic distress and disquietude, gripping his muscles to the bones of his body, without him even realizing it. "Sure," he says.

"What is her name?"

"Her name?"

"Yes, sir."

"Oh, yes, yes . . . it's uh . . . Jo . . . Jo . . . Jolene Marie Walker. Yes. Jolene Marie Walker."

"Can you spell her first name for me?"

Mosiah sighs and then begins to spell out Jolene's name. He listens and answers the receptionist's questions: Does she have insurance? Has she had any other symptoms besides the suspicious body pimple? What day would she like to come for her appointment? What time? Has she ever been to the Mayo campus before? Mosiah answers each question more emboldened by his actions with every response. He waves Donald away from the door while he finishes up on the phone. Donald closes the door to the office. The meeting of the edge of the door with the frame, pulls the rest of the air out of the room. Mosiah coughs into the receiver.

"Sir, are you alright?"

"Yes," he ekes out. "A breeze caught me the wrong way."

"Well, I hope you feel better. The appointment for your wife is all set. We'll see her the Tuesday after Memorial Day."

"Thank you," Mosiah says.

The woman hangs up her end of the call. Mosiah holds the phone to his ear for a moment before realizing she is gone. He is done. He looks at the screen the white screen, of the keypad, and closes it.

Might as well tell Jo.

He texts her:

> Your appointment is Tuesday May 29.
> At Mayo Clinic.
>   What appointment?
> You know what I'm talking about.
> I just made it.
> Saved you the trouble.

Mosiah stares at the phone, waiting to see what message the blinking, animated ellipses will turn into. He waits to see if she will send an angry emoji, a bitmoji caricature of herself saying "WTF," or a GIF of a frightened baby, or neck rolling reality star, questioning his actions. None of that comes. The ellipses go away, then come back again. They go away and come back again. He can tell she's typing responses and deleting them over and over again, processing her feelings for what he's done, and for how she wants to react to what he's done. At one in the afternoon, he knows she can't cause a scene because she's teaching, and she can't step out of the classroom for too long without reason. Any other time, she would have called by now, but she can't. He watches the phone, waiting to see how angry she is. It finally vibrates and whistles in his hand. One word. Not even. One letter. "K." Mosiah releases another breath he didn't know he was holding. He rolls away from the desk shoved up against the wall, and stands up. Dropping the phone in his back pocket, he hits the light to the office, and walks out onto the barbershop floor.

"Donald, did you need me for something?" he asks, taking a seat in his chair.

"Nah, man, I'm good," Donald says. "Was just checking on you. That's all. You disappeared. That's unlike you."

"We're not too busy in here, and I have a lil' minute before my next client. I just had to handle something, that's all."

"What for?" Bobby asks from behind him.

"Damn, man, you nosy," Ryan says.

Mosiah laughs. Donald and Bobby were always the loudest and the most outgoing in the shop. Chris and Ryan were typically quiet. Both jumping into conversations only when they had something to add. They jumped out just as quickly as the discussions ebbed and flowed around three main topics: money, women, and sports. All four were fiercely loyal to Mosiah and just as protective. Ryan, moreso, guarded Mosiah's inner man from Bobby, who felt privy and entitled to all parts of him, because they'd known each other the longest.

"It's alright," Mosiah says to Ryan. "I had to make an appointment for Jolene to see the doctor."

"For what?" Bobby asks again.

"Now you're being nosy," Mosiah says.

Donald says, "You need to get you some business, man, and stop minding everybody else's."

"Mo, is like my brother," Bobby defends.

"And there are some things even brothers don't share," Ryan says.

"Exactly," Mosiah cosigns.

"Especially about their wives," Ryan says.

Ryan was the only other married man in the shop. A newlywed, married just two years ago. His wedding was a massive affair in Orlando, Mosiah and Jolene attended at the JW Marriott Grande Lakes. Mosiah knew the family of Ryan's wife paid for the wedding, but Ryan never let it bother him. He said, "If they want to spend all their money and go into debt to give her away to me, that's on them. I know what I have, and she knows what she's coming into."

Since the wedding, Ryan began getting to the shop early, the same time Mosiah arrived, to help him open up, and he stayed late to help Mosiah close down and clean up. He picked up any early morning, or last minute walk-ins along the way. Ryan put his wedding band on a silver chain when he walked in, to keep it from getting dirty or tarnished by the creams and cleansers he used to cut hair. In its place, around his finger was a tattoo of a thin wedding band, on his neck, his wife's name, Fatima, and on his left arm were their vows, tatted in ink for anyone to see he was off the market and off-limits to any other woman. The visual cues were helpful to the single mother's who brought their sons into the shop for haircuts, and the few girls with bald fades, and short natural cuts, who preferred a man to keep them edged and shaped up, over a woman.

"Thanks, man," Mosiah says, giving Ryan a head nod.

"That's some next level love," Roger, one of Chris's regulars, says from the chair. "You making appointments for your wife and what not."

"Not really," Mosiah says. "She didn't have time. I did. It ain't nothing."

"That's what husbands do," Ryan says.

"How long y'all been married, man?" Gary, the client in Donald's chair, asks.

"Six going on seven years," Mosiah answers.

"Y'all for real family now," Roger says.

"We've been family since before we got together," Mosiah says. "Me putting a ring on her finger just took it to a whole 'nother level."

Mosiah spins in his chair away from his barbers and their clients. Facing the mirror, his hands in his lap, he fondles the so-called meteorite wedding band on his finger. The ring Jolene found for him online, allegedly made from an authentic meteorite, a piece of dinosaur bone, and yellow gold. She slid it on his finger as she recited her memorized vows, splicing them in with the traditional ones given by his father, the preacher. She said, "With this ring, I thee wed, my soulmate with whom I will walk through the cold. I gift you gold, a precious metal your heart outshines. I gird you with the rock of ancient bones, because from the first man until the last, there is no one else for me. And last, but not least, I encircle you with a touch of meteorite, for you are the stuff of what the world is made of, in whom I will always delight.

"Mo, is what they say true?" Ryan asks, just above the raucous of the men in the shop.

"Is what true?" Mo asks, spinning toward him.

"You know. When you reach seven years. Is it true?"

"I'm not there yet?"

"Are you itching to leave?" Donald asks.

"Leave who?" Mosiah asks. "My wife? Hell nah."

"Then it's not true," Donald reasons toward Ryan.

"I didn't say that," Mosiah says. "I'm just saying, I'm not leaving my wife. We have ups and downs. And sometimes it's just middle ground. We just chug along in the middle of the road, but we know what we have; and I ain't going nowhere, and she ain't going nowhere, even if we do get on each other's last fucking nerve sometime."

"That's real," Ryan says.

"Why? You and Fatima beefin'?"

"Nah," Ryan answers. He spins his client toward the mirror and talks with his back toward Mosiah. "Nothing like that. Just asking."

Mosiah says, "When I proposed. I meant forever. For me there is no divorce. Just death do us part."

The men in the shop don't respond to Mosiah's declaration of his definition of love and marriage, in terms of his relationship. He spins back toward the mirror, his mind on the day he proposed.

He was standing under the portico at one of the designated picnic areas at Hanna Park; the park that offered nature walks, bike trails, and most importantly, access to the beach. That's where Jolene surprised him with a barbecue to celebrate his graduation, and one year of the shop being open. A sign hung between two of the awning posts that said "Congratulations, Mo." His parents were there, her parents, and sisters, and grandmother, the barbers from the shop, and a host of other people milled around, eating plates of ribs and baked beans, burgers and potato salad, macaroni and cheese and chicken leg quarters, slathered in sauce. She told him they were going to a barbecue. What she didn't tell him was that she was throwing him a barbecue.

He arrived excited and embarrassed, the ring he bought two weeks earlier burning a hole through his right hand, that he kept shoved in his pocket to clutch the velvet box that would decide their fate. As the barbecue wound down, Jolene took his hand and led him toward the sand. He followed her lead after looking back at her father, and giving him a knowing nod. He'd asked Mr. Lewis for her hand in marriage shortly after her graduation. He sought out approval and confirmation before buying the ring nearly six months earlier; just weeks after she first found out he was home, by their happenstance meeting in the barbershop. When they pulled up to the party and he saw all the faces gathered for him, he knew it was time to let her in on the plan he'd had from the moment she left his shop when she accidentally, or by sublime coincidence, found him for good.

On the beach, they walked the hard packed sand of the sea floor at low tide, arm in arm, admiring the crush of the ocean beneath the pull of the rising moon, and the setting sun. The words they exchanged were few. Their conversation was mostly that of mood and emotion. She tugged, he leaned, they walked together, in step, hands held, fingers intertwined, heads inclined toward the other. It wasn't until Mosiah could hear the murmurs of excited chatter, and feel the dozen or more sets of eyes on his back, that he guided an oblivious Jolene back the way they came. He guided her from the hard sand, to the soft sinking sand that sticks to your skin and in the crevices between your toes. Mosiah waited until Jolene was veering toward the access ramp to rejoin her family who waited, seemingly nonplussed, just out of reach of the dunes. They were far enough away for them to extend privacy, but still close enough to see the inevitable expressions of love.

As Jolene began to struggle to get Mosiah to keep her pace, he fell to all fours. He blamed it on a root he stumbled over. Jolene rushed to his side to help him up, but as she stood, holding and tugging his hand, he remained on the ground, holding just one of hers. When she finally realized what was happening, and stopped asking, "What are you doing?" "Are you sure you're okay?" "Did you sprain an ankle or something?" "Are you okay?" he was halfway done with his proposal.

Tears streamed down her face and blurred her sight as she began to make excuses for why she couldn't except his proposal, why she couldn't say yes, why he shouldn't even be down on both knees, presenting her a ring. "What about Toussaint?" "I have a kid." "You know you can find somebody better than me." "Somebody that doesn't have all this baggage." "I thought we were just friends."

To that he said, "We're a whole lot more than friends and you know it. We have been since we were three."

Jolene blubbered her way through more excuses. Mosiah shut down each and every one until she collapsed in his arms, kissed his top lip, and finally said yes. Mosiah slid the two carat diamond held by white gold, on her finger, picked her up in his arms as he stood from the sand, and carried her the rest of the way up the beach, and back to the picnic area where their family and friends waited.

"So Mo," Ryan says, interrupting Mosiah's trance. "If you had to do it all over again, would you?"

"In a heartbeat."

"You said you're going on seven years, right?" Chris asks.

"Yup," Mosiah answers. "Next March will make seven years."

"Then maybe you should do it all over," Chris suggests. "Like a vow renewal ceremony."

"For seven years?" Mosiah scoffs. "Most people don't do that until they get to like twenty-five years."

"Most marriages these days don't last twenty-five years," Ryan says.

"Yeah, what's the average?" Bobby asks. "Like six, eight years."

"Something like that," Donald says.

"I'm just saying," Ryan adds. "If next year is lucky number seven, and you ain't itching to leave, it won't hurt to do it all over again."

"You know they say seven is a divine number," Roger says as Chris dusts him off.

"I know," Mosiah says. "My old man says it all the time."

"That's right, church boy," Bobby says. "Then you should know better than anybody how lucky seven is."

"I know, I know," Mosiah says. "The number of completion. The number of alignment. The number of becoming. I know."

"I'm just saying it could be a good anniversary gift for JoJo," Bobby says. "Nothing says I love you forever, than to redo the moment you made the commitment in the first place."

Mosiah spins to look at Bobby who also sits in his chair. With a raised eyebrow he says, "Look at you, Mr. I'm Never Getting Married In My Life. When did you all of a sudden become the champion of love and commitments?"

"I'm not saying I want to get married," Bobby says. "I got my own issues. But that shit works for guys like you and Ryan. I'm just trying to support."

"Guys like me and Ryan?" Mosiah repeats.

"Yeah, Bobby," Ryan says. "What the hell is that supposed to mean?"

"It just means y'all the family man, settling down type," Donald says, defending Bobby. "Chris is too."

"And where does that leave you and Bobby?" Chris asks.

"To roam wild and free for as long as can be," Bobby says.

"My man," Donald agrees.

"If you don't feel free in your marriage, you married the wrong woman," Roger says. "I'll check y'all later."

The bell above the door rings with his exit.

"One time for the old head dropping knowledge on his way out," Bobby says.

The rest of the men nod their agreement. Mosiah turns away from Bobby and looks in the mirror. He sees exhaustion in his eyes, even though he's not tired. The stress of Jolene's hemming and hawing about her own health, weighs on him. Mosiah sighs and closes his eyes in his chair. He takes a few breaths, hoping a few moments of meditation will at least clear his face, even if it doesn't automatically clear his mind.

He picked up meditation in the military. There were only so many times he could re-read the latest letter from his mom, his dad, Jolene, or a few select others, before he'd memorized their words. There were only so many times he could write new replies before his hand cramped from holding a pen. He tried to sleep away whatever idle time he had, but he couldn't. His body was trained, regimented, and scheduled to only shut down when it was lights out, and not a moment before. During his down time, he took to sitting or laying with his eyes closed, focused on nothing but the audible sound of his breath, until he could hear his heart beat and feel it slowing down as it took less effort to pump blood through his relaxed body.

Do it all over again. That could be nice. Better than the first time.

Mosiah opens his eyes. He sees clarity in the whites of his sclera, convinced to make the second time around better than the first. The first time, they didn't have much money. It was the reason they got married in the small church Mosiah grew up in. The church his father pastored. Sweet Love of Christ AME. Their family and friends packed the pews in the small sanctuary, compared to the mega-church

Jolene attended that was a few streets away. They couldn't afford her mega-church or its pastor, so Reverend Paul Alan Walker performed their ceremony, Granny Mae catered the reception, and he and Jolene took what they had to pay for the venue that was in the middle of a rundown strip mall. The most activity in the area came from the liquor store across the parking lot, with the tall sign that could be seen and read from the highway, even if half of its electric lights were busted or burnt out.

Doing it again wouldn't be so bad. We could do it the way we really want to this time.

Mosiah wipes his hands over his face, trying to swipe away the stress resting in his countenance. He brushes one hand over the back of his low cut hair, while the other fondles the square trim of his goatee that hangs below his chin. He brings his hands to rest over his mouth and nose, two fingers steepled between his eyes. He nods to himself in the mirror.

Let's do it again.

Maybe this way she won't be so mad at me about calling the doctor.

"Jo, you home?" Mosiah yells as he opens the door to the quiet house.

"Upstairs," he hears her yell.

Mosiah kicks off his work boots and jogs up the flight of stairs to find Jolene. His pace is bolstered by the excitement of telling her he wants to get remarried, of proposing again, of choosing her all over again. The idea grew stronger within him throughout the day after Ryan's initial suggestion. His mind jumped from having a wedding on the beach, to having a wedding on the river bank in St. Augustine. He picked colors, chose his best man, and had come up with a menu and a theme by the time he and Ryan closed the shop for the night. On his drive to the news station he decided against calling the foremen of the cleaning crews he had heading up jobs at three other commercial properties across the city, and instead, let his mind wander as

Jill Scott and Anthony Hamilton serenaded him about being so in love.

He sang along to the latest staple in the catalogue of black wedding songs until the track changed, and he was bombarded by the heavenly arrangement of an O'Jay's sample with the coarse voice of a jazz singer turned hipster. Mosiah sang every track on the playlist of love songs he'd made for him and Jolene, leading up to their wedding. The mix of male and female R&B singers kept him energized as he vacuumed, wiped, dusted, polished, mopped, and made small talk with the few people in the cavernous news building. He and the crew finished early, and instead of being the last one of his guys to drive out of the parking lot of the new job, he was the first. He peeled down the empty downtown streets, crossed the red Mathews Bridge, and headed home with his windows down, his music up, and his own harmony nearly drowning out the voices, the music, the bass, and the melody pumping out of his sound system. Most men put subwoofers in their cars to bang the bass as loud as possible on their favorite hip-hop or rock song. Mosiah put a subwoofer in his extended cab, midnight blue F-150 because he liked his music loud, and the subtle but steady bass of traditional R&B filled his soul with song.

At the top of the stairs, Mosiah peaks in on Lydia and Toussaint in their rooms. Lydia was asleep beneath Princess Tiana covers. Her body is half off the bed. He sees her feet pointing down to the ground, as if she were going to slide off the bed and stand up at attention. Mosiah adjusts her so that she is under the covers. Her frog humidifier blows a steady stream of filtered mist and vapor into the air that clouds her face in an angelic halo of dew. Mosiah walks back toward the door and closes it behind him. In Toussaint's room, the scene is everything but calm. Clothes are scattered across his bed and on the carpeted floor. He lays back on his bed, his head against the wall, a complicated video controller in his hand. Mosiah pushes the door open to his room and walks in front of the small nineteen-inch flat screen, mounted in a corner in the room obstructing his view. He can see

Toussaint's delayed response to his presence. His leaning from side to side to see around Mosiah's body.

"Turn the game off and go to bed," Mosiah says. "It's a school night."

"I'm playing until I lose," Toussaint says, still leaning and weaving to see his game.

Mosiah turns around and hits the power button on the game system and the television.

"Mo . . . C'mon . . ." Toussaint whines.

"You lose. Go to bed."

"Okaaaayyyyy . . ." Toussaint huffs.

He kicks more clothes to the floor as he thrashes his body under the covers. "Good night," he says, pulling the comforter over his head.

"Tomorrow you're going to clean this room," Mosiah says. "You've got shit everywhere."

"Okkkaaayyyy . . ."

"I could never keep my room as filthy as you keep yours. I don't know why your mama let you live like this in the first place."

"Good night, Mo," Toussaint says.

"You can't put me out of no room in *my* house, TeeTee." Mosiah says. "This is my house."

"I know," Toussaint says through gritting teeth.

"Don't turn that game back on, TeeTee. Turn it on and I will tear it down."

"Okkkkkaaayyyy . . ."

Mosiah walks out of Toussaint's room and closes the door. He waits beside it to see if he hears the power to the television cut back on. With his ear pressed to the door, he waits just a few seconds before finally walking away from Toussaint's closed door, into his own room. Inside, he finds Jolene naked, sitting on the their lilac sheets rubbing lotion into her body.

"Well, damn," Mosiah says, closing and locking the door behind him. "I can get used to coming home like this."

"Boy, hush," Jolene says, laughing. "I just got out the tub when you walked in the door yelling, and I didn't see no reason in covering up since Lydia's asleep and Toussaint was playing that damn game."

You should have made him go to sleep.

"Ain't no need in you covering up nothing. I already seen what you got."

"Mmmhmmm."

"Outside and inside." Mosiah flicks his tongue in an obscene gesture.

"Stop being mannish."

"You know you like it."

"I never said I didn't."

"I know. That's what I thought," Mosiah says, crossing the room to where Jolene sits. He kisses her on her forehead. "I'm going take a shower."

Mosiah hums one of the songs from his playlist as he pulls off his work suit. The one about being a fool for the one he loves. In the shower, Mosiah keeps humming. He transitions from the song about fools in love, to one about how loving another person is more than just a dream come true. Mosiah hums the soprano key in his adept tenor as he soaps his body. He hangs up the towel and places the soap back in the caddy, before turning the water off and stepping out of the lukewarm shower, the majority of the hot water he figures went to her bath.

Dripping water across the bathroom floor, Mosiah walks naked into the bedroom where Jolene is now in her long-sleeved crop top night-shirt with the words "spoil me" written in large block letters across her unrestrained breasts. She wears just the shirt and underwear. The comforter and top sheet are barely pulled up to her navel, giving Mosiah easy access to stare at the skin she didn't cover. One leg is wrapped on top of the comforter, helping to regulate her body temperature, and giving him a view of her voluptuous thighs.

"I had an idea today," Mosiah says, pulling out blue plaid boxers from the chest of the drawers.

"Oh yeah?" Jolene encourages. "What was that?"

"What would you say if I said we should get married again?"

"I'd say you were crazy."

"That's it."

"No. You didn't let me finish."

"Ah . . . Okay."

"But I'd also say let's do it again."

"How about for our anniversary next year?"

"That's wildly specific and soon."

"I know."

"You really want to plan a wedding in eight months?"

Mosiah slides into the bed beside Jolene. "It's not a wedding, just a vow renewal."

"Same thing."

"We can do it," Mosiah insists.

"Then we have to start planning now," Jolene says talking faster. "We have to pick a location, and get a caterer, I need a new dress . . ."

"We already have a date."

"I know. March ninth. I think I can lose thirty pounds by then."

"Thirty?"

"Yes. Thirty."

"You don't need to lose an inch."

"Thank you. But I am too damn big and you know it."

"Not at all."

Mosiah grabs the thickness of Jolene's thigh and squeezes it until she squeals and rolls away from him. He uses his arm to gather her back to him until they are nose to nose.

"Good night."

He kisses her nose and her lips, then reaches behind him to turn off the lamp on the nightstand.

"I love you," he says, once he's facing her again.

"I love you too," Jolene says.

He holds on to her waist as her body settles in the bed. In the darkness of their room he watches her as he did when he was a toddler. She yawns, her eyes blink rapidly, and then they close. He watches as slumber overtakes her etching peace into her visage. The skin of her face is dewy from her nighttime moisturizer and serene in its silence. Gone are the worry lines that wrinkle her brow when she is contemplative about something, removed are the questions and uncertainty that often cloud her eyes during the day, as she struggles to determine if she's made the right decisions. He looks down on her lips, her ripe and supple mouth that, even though it is unsmiling, is still inviting. The bow shape, with the pink tint is still an invitation to him that he is welcome to all of her.

Mosiah leans in and kisses just her lips.

With her eyes still closed she asks, "You really want to marry me again?"

"If I could do it all over again every day of my life, I would say yes to you every day of my life."

Thank you. "Thank you," Jolene says aloud.

"For what?" Mosiah asks.

"For loving me the way that you do." *Even when I don't deserve it.*

"You're easy to love."

Even when I want to push him away, I can't. "Thank you," Jolene says.

This time she leans forward and kisses Mosiah. First his nose and then his lips. He doesn't let her retreat. He holds her tighter still to his body and kisses her back. He kisses her with the full force of the passion his idea stoked inside him since that afternoon in the shop. He savors her lips and caresses her tongue with his own. Mosiah's arm tightens around Jolene's waist until the soft, warmth of her body is prostrate against him. He pulls the full force of her weight on top of him. She doesn't stop kissing him as her hands stroke the stubble of his cheek and smooths over the top of his hair.

His hands work to remove her underwear. She follows his lead, sliding his boxers down off of his hips. He lifts his pelvis, with her still sitting astride him, in the air to fully remove the boxers. His hands find her ass and squeeze. They run up the sides of her waist beneath her shirt to her breasts, barely contained by the sweatshirt material overlaying them. Mosiah holds on to Jolene as he sits up straight in the bed. She wraps her legs around the back of his naked waist as he reclines against the pillow soft headboard.

He breaks their kiss to oblige the message on her shirt and spoil her breasts. With two hands he brings each one to his mouth and kisses first, her brown nipples the color of candied walnuts. He savors them as Jolene rocks her wetness against his stiffness, longing to connect their bodies the way they connected their mouths. He kisses, licks, and suckles her breast as she rocks her way through her first orgasm. Her release coats his dick, hips, and thighs and makes it easy for him to slide right into her nirvana. His hands run up the sides of her body, pulling the sweatshirt over her head and her scarf right along with it. Her thick hair begins to fall out of its protective wrap as he pulls her waist even closer into his, with every stroke through her inner sanctum. He claims her mouth as he claims her body. The orb of his extension strokes consistently in the caverns she's offered, trying to find new depths, new sensations, and new pleasures.

Jolene reaches behind Mosiah and grabs the top of the headboard for balance. She unwraps her legs from around his waist and brings them beside her, until her knees are pressed into the top of the bed. Using the headboard as leverage, she rides him slow, forwards and backwards, side to side, up and down. She works him from every angle until his hands find her waist to try to increase her pace. Gripping the headboard with her hands and his legs with her knees, she makes her movements short and succint. Jolene drops her bottom and all it's ancestral weight on him again and again, until she's forced to pull to the apex of his penis, before slamming into his base to allow yet another of her releases flow.

Mosiah rears his hips and pushes her backward onto the bed. He grabs one of her legs and flips her over, and then pulls her back into him, so he can slide into her. His fingers grip the inner creases leading to her essence and pull until he is positioned with purpose in her expanse. He pumps into her with the electric energy he had when she first offered herself to him in this way. Both of them well past virginity, they were still awkward and shy fumbling over each other's bodies as their friendship fast-forwarded past the point of no return. He pumps into her, remembering their first time when his excitement overcame him and he had to apologize for not meeting his own expectations. He pumps into her in full control of his own body, his own intentions, and his own gratification destination.

Jolene grips the fitted sheet on the bed and flexes her feet behind her. She pulls herself to her knees, but leaves her chest and arms flat across the bed. She rolls her lower body into him with his every pull, sending a ripple of waves from her diaphragm into his own body. She meets his force with force until he lays completely over her body. Their knees thrash and clash on the sheets. She turns her face to meet his for a kiss, another connection, and the first undoing of his bold erection. She sucks his tongue, bites his bottom lip, and smothers his face again with her passion until he has to pull back. She overwhelms his mouth so much, he has to retreat to focus on his phallus.

Jolene reaches for his hands, bringing his body forward onto hers once more. She intertwines the fingers of their right hand as he moves his left hand down the parted sea of her breast, over the mound of her mommy tummy, and to top of their congruent connection. Guiding his fingers to where she wants them, he finds the space where he has to peel back the layers to tickle her bundled ivory.

Mosiah moves their bodies to the center of the bed and then lays down on his side. He strokes Jolene from behind, while patting the center of her sensuality until it throbs beneath his digital power, for the release he's been denying himself.

Jolene turns her face toward the hand she's holding and kisses the center of his right palm. His left pats her pound as she works her tongue up from the base of his middle finger, the entire time his stroke never stops. It increases in power as his strumming hand works in tandem to uncork the heavy flow she can no longer hold inside. Jolene lets her body burst with pleasure and exhale with sensation as she squeezes Mosiah's fingers between her jaws, sucking them until her cheeks pops. She flows around him and then rolls her body back onto the bed. She lays prostrate on the soaked sheets as Mosiah rears behind her once more, working quickly into her body before she comes down from the high he created. He bangs his way past inhibitions, putting his prowess at the center of the exhibition to be judged, in the only language of approval he cares to hear.

Her muffled moans turn into buried screams as she tries to wrench her body away from him and he pulls her back into his passion. With one final thrust, he gives in to temptation and lets the pent up passion send ecstasy through his sweat wet body, as it sends life into hers. The reverberation of his release stirs in her deep, and ignites a gush of her own gluttony to drench him as he drenched her.

Mosiah collapses on top of Jolene. His chest to her back. His heart beating through to her skin, her heart beating into the bed. They exhale deeply from their nose as the fog of phantasm disappears, and they become aware of the cool air from the AC working overtime in the humidity of their embodied homes. Jolene sighs in a humming moan as exhaustion from her exertion overcomes her.

It's moments like this when I know I'm never leaving. I just need to get out of my own head.

"C'mon," Mosiah says, scooting them away from the wet spot they created.

On the dry side of the bed, Mosiah pulls the top sheet and then the comforter over them cocooning their cooling bodies, creating heat once again. Jolene expels him from her body and rolls over to face him.

"Good night."

"Good night," Mosiah says.

He watches her fall asleep as he always does. He is no longer on a cot away from her but right beside her, where he knew he always belonged. His hand resting on her breast, his fingers avoid finding what he knows is there. He lays there in blissful ignorance, willing his mind to forget the fact that there is something between them that could change them.

Change her. He lays there and watches her sleep, unwilling to see the images he searched online in her body. He lays there watching her chest, her legs, her arms, all of her rise and fall with life, with breath, with vibrancy, and with the soul of their love. He watches her with his lids forced open, not knowing what is to come, only that he will love her forever.

We're going to make it, he promises himself. *We're going to do it over.*

Mosiah sighs and falls asleep humming a song he sang earlier. The song composed with lilting strings and a flowing melody that builds up into the crescendo of the chorus. The lyrics are his plea, his prayer to the God his father raised him to serve.

Lord, I'm not asking for much. Just a couple of forevers.

He hums himself to sleep, turning the R&B words into his petition for what he's seen to be a lie, and for what he's felt to be benign.

11.

"Mrs. Walker, what brings you in today?" Doctor Araya Richards asks.

"I've been dizzy and lightheaded lately, and I have been having a pain in my side," Jolene says.

She sits on the cushioned paper-covered table in the cold exam room, with her jeans still on and a pink paper top covering her breasts and belly. Her waist trainer is sitting in the lone chair, behind the privacy curtain, off to the side of the room, and her Spanx are rolled down under her fat. There is no window to the outside world from the exam room in the premiere hospital. She sits facing an ecru wall with a clock, and a mounted Plexiglas pamphlet holder containing trifold medical literature on everything from childbirth to ovarian cancer.

"Are those the only symptoms you've been having?" Doctor Richards asks?

"Yes."

"It says here, on your new patient intake form, that you were concerned about a spot on your breast?"

"It's not a spot, and it's not on my breast?" Jolene says. "It's underneath. Like on my skin."

"Let's take a look and see what's going on. Lay back for me."

Jolene does as she's told and lays down. The paper of her pink top crunches against the paper of the exam table. She lays down and stairs at the drywall tiled ceiling as Dr. Richards examines her chest. One cold hand lifts, pokes, and prods the left breast, and then the right breast. Jolene avoids making eye contact with the spectacled woman whose ethnicity she cannot immediately identify. She stares at the top of her head, where the mushroom bobbed cut hair with bangs falls from its shape, hovers over her chest, and allows her to see the doctor's alabaster scalp.

She's taking longer on this side than she did the other one.

"Is everything alright?" Jolene asks.

"Seems to be."

"How long have you had that mole?" Dr. Richards asks. "You can sit up."

Jolene heaves her body forward. She closes up the open paper vest and looks at the doctor. She studies her face waiting for her to render a verdict on her health. Doctor Richards stares right back. Her pale face, dark hair, and stark white lab coat give nothing away.

She asks again, "How long have you had that mole?"

"A month, maybe more," Jolene says.

"Was it always hard like that?"

"I guess. I don't inspect it everyday. I thought it was just like any other mole."

"Do you have other moles on your body?"

"No. Not really. More beauty marks than anything else. There's one between my toes. One on my collarbone. This one here on my middle finger."

Jolene holds up her left hand and spreads her finger for Doctor Richards to see the random marking on one part of her body, superstition signifies as beautiful. The doctor doesn't come close to inspect it. She stays standing, an arms length away, feet firmly planted on the ground, body upright and rigid in front of the countertop and sink.

"That's different, Mrs. Walker. Those beauty marks by comparison are inconsequential to the mole beneath your breast. Could be nothing but I think you should get it biopsied just to be safe."

"Is that absolutely necessary?" Jolene asks. "I have other moles on my body. Look at my neck."

Jolene strains and cranes her neck for Doctor Richards' benefit. Again, she does not come close to see.

"Those moles are smaller. Tiny in fact," Dr. Richards says. "What's on your skin is different in shape, size, and texture. Feel it."

Doctor Richards waits for Jolene to examine her own body. To know herself as well as she claims she does. Jolene moves her manicured hands into the open paper top and feels for the pimple-like mole protruding from her skin.

"Okay," she says.

"What does it feel like?" Doctor Richards asks.

"Feels like a mole."

"Besides that."

"Like a red bean, the way it's hard and shaped."

"Exactly," Doctor Richards says, her face just as blasé and her voice as equally staid as before. "That's not normal, you need to have it checked. A biopsy would be the best way."

"Not a mammogram?" Jolene asks. "That's what I thought I was here for?"

"We can do a mammogram, but if the results are inconclusive, we'd have to do an ultrasound and a biopsy anyway."

"How long will it take for that?" Jolene asks.

"Go to the front and make an appointment. They should get you back in here within at least a couple weeks, if you don't have any scheduling conflicts."

I guess. I don't know why everyone thinks something is wrong with me. I would know if I was sick with something.

"I'll see you in a few weeks," Doctor Richards says, not waiting for an affirmative answer.

"But what about my dizziness, headaches, and shortness of breath?" Jolene asks.

"I'll write you a prescription, just in case it's vertigo. But the best medicine for that is rest. I still want that mole biopsied."

Doctor Richards pulls her prescription pad out of her coat pocket and scribbles on it. Jolene watches her tear the paper and toss it on top of the counter, before walking out of the exam room. The door closes behind her. Jolene sees the scrip and the file Doctor Richards left. She slides off the cushion counter and steps down from the table. Pulling back the privacy curtain Jolene stands in front of the mirror and pulls the pink paper vest off of her shoulders. Her breasts lay heavy against her skin. She lifts the right one, the offending boob, and looks at the small protrusion. It is only slightly darker than her praline complexion. She pulls it away from her body and squeezes it. Nothing comes out. Not puss, not blood, not even what she initially thought was an ingrown hair.

Maybe a biopsy won't be so bad. I still don't understand what this has to do with me being tired and dizzy and achy. I probably just need a massage. Mo spending money at this fancy ass hospital, knowing good and damn well my insurance ain't this good. I could have gone to the urgent clinic for all she did. They probably would have told me what I already know. This is nothing to worry about and I just need to eat right, exercise, and sleep so I can stop being so dizzy and tired. I need a vacation, but Lord knows he won't leave that shop, or stop cleaning up after people for no long period of time.

Me, Tanya, and Vaughn could take a girls trip. That would be nice. We've never done that.

Jolene fastens her bra around her body then spins the tangerine, lace demi-cup contraption, until it is facing the right direction. She pulls it over her arms and shoves the fatty tissue that wants to spill out of its restraint deep inside, so that just a bit more than her nipples are covered by the undergarment she should have given up two cup sizes ago. Jolene jumps as she rolls up her body shaper before pulling her loose orange V-neck blouse over her head. It falls over her body and floats away from her skin. She adjusts the bottom hem of the shirt until the front and back pieces lay in a way she's satisfied with over her belly, and tucked just enough in the crease of her back to show off her butt. Feet into sandals, purse on her arm, Jolene shoves the waist trainer deep into the gold bag, and slings it over her shoulder as she takes one last look in the mirror.

The weight gain hasn't been all bad.

She admires her perfect apple bottom for a few more seconds. Her sandals slap the tile of the floor as she snatches her medical file from the countertop and flings open the door of the exam room. The manila folder with her most personal information, financial and otherwise, swishes back and forth against her thigh as she walks to the checkout counter. There is no line when she arrives. She slides the folder to the receptionist and waits, allowing her mind to wander over what she will do with her free time.

I might as well as enjoy the rest of the day off before I have to get Lydia and Toussaint. I could go shopping. Get some bigger clothes, because these jeans are holding on for dear life; cutting all into my fat, even with the Spanx. Mo watched me get dressed this morning, talking 'bout, "What you need all that for?" Because I need it. Damn.

"We can get you in for your biopsy on Wednesday, June thirteenth at 9 a.m.," the receptionist says, looking from the computer to Jolene.

"That's fine."

"Do. You need an appointment card?"

"No. I'll put it in my phone. Have a good day," Jolene says, walking away from the woman's desk.

Jolene pushes the door out of the office and into the hallway with her shoulder. She drops one strap of her purse and reaches inside the open mouth for her phone. She calls Vaughn as she opts to take the stairs down to the ground floor of the building, and out to the parking lot.

"This is Vaughn," her sister answers on the third ring.

"Whatchu doin'?" Jolene asks.

"Working, Jo. Like you should be doing."

"I have the day off," Jolene says.

"For what?" Vaughn asks.

"Mo made me come to the doctor for this small-ass mole on my stomach."

"Mo made you go to the doctor?" Vaughn asks, her voice rising. "For a mole?"

"That's what I said. But you know Mo. Once he gets an idea in his head, he ain't letting it go."

"No, he's only that way with you. He don't want nothing to happen to his precious Jolene."

"I keep telling that man I'm not a porcelain doll. I'm not going to break. But he keeps smothering me like I'm not his already."

"I think it's sweet. Most women would kill to have they man still sweatin' them after they've been married the way Mo is with you."

"Then you'll really love this," Jolene says. "He said he wants to renew our vows for our anniversary next year."

"Are you serious?" Vaughn asks squealing.

"Girl, yes."

"Oh my gosh. I can't wait. Another wedding. Girl, we gotta go shopping and get you a dress. Meet me in San Marco."

"Right now, Vaughn?" Jolene asks.

"Yes, right now. You said you're off for the rest of the day."

"I know *I* am, but aren't you working?" Jolene asks, getting into her SUV.

"Yes, but I can leave if I want to. I'm the Senior Marketing Specialist. As long as I'm reachable, I'm technically working."

"Fine, but I still have to cross the bridge. It's gon' be a minute."

"That's fine. I can sit here and pretend like I'm working like I've been doing all day anyway. What's another twenty minutes?"

"Wish I had it made like you," Jolene says wistfully, as she pulls out into the light traffic on San Pablo Road.

"Everybody ain't able," Vaughn says. "Call me when you're getting ready to get off on 95."

"For what? Just meet me on wedding row in front of the old La Nopalera in twenty minutes."

"Jo, I swear you act like you got a minute phone."

Jolene laughs. "I do."

"You know good and damn well they don't even make those anymore."

"Just meet me over there in the parking lot."

"I will."

Jolene hears the phone line go silent. Immediately, music comes through the stereo. Heavy trap beats lay the foundation; a choir later covers with harmonies and melodies and lyrics that uplift. Jolene turns the music down. The sudden loud noise makes her head hurt. She resists the urge to put her head on the steering wheel, even though her eyesight blurs momentarily, and the SUV shifts and swerves under her uncontrollable power. It takes, what feels like minutes, but is only seconds to course correct and even out the truck. Cars on her right and left blow by her after she's straightened up. They lay on their horns well after they've passed her, their necks still craning backwards to look Jolene in the face, so she will remember their grimaces. It is the behavior of passive aggressive people. The people everyone becomes behind the wheel of any motorized machine. The people who ride bumpers, flash their lights, fishtail in and out of lanes, and cut one another off. Jolene is thankful all she got were grimaces instead of the select special few who make defensive driving a hunting sport, where the offended or even the offenders, take it upon themselves to shoot their prey when there was no reason to kill.

It's one in the afternoon and everybody is pissed off already.

Jolene moves into the right lane and continues on the state road that will take her to the interstate.

I don't even know why I let Vaughn talk me into this. I should have just gone to pick up Lydia early, and then came back to grab Toussaint. Or stopped by the shop to see Mo. I know he's dying to know what happened at my appointment today. Well, he should have been there when I went since he made it. But no, he didn't want Ryan or Bobby left alone trying to run the shop. I don't understand the point of having employees and other barbers, if he's not going to trust them to do what needs to be done if he's not there. He can't be there all the time, but Lord knows he tries. That's why we barely take vacations as it is. Hell, that's what we should do for our anniversary next year. Forget a vow renewal. We should finally have a real honeymoon, instead of that staycation bullshit we did the first time. I want to go somewhere far. Get stamps in my passport. Hell, I need to get a passport first. Mo's been all over the world, might as well do it together now.

Jolene feels the smile creeping across her face and her body warming with thoughts of blue water and white sand, on tropical vacations. She gets off I-95 before crossing the Main Street Bridge and takes Prudential Drive to Hendricks Avenue, until she is between the recently vacated building of the infamous Mexican restaurant on her left, and block after block of boutiques dedicated to all things bridal on her right.

Jolene pulls into the parking lot and finds a spot beside Vaughn's beat-up yellow Bug.

"Hurry up. Let's go," Vaughn yells after Jolene cuts the engine.

Jolene glares at Vaughn through the window of her car. Her sister leans against the door of the five-year-old Beetle, dressed in a purple romper with black breast pockets and lace up sandals. The cuff of the romper is pulled nearly to her knee to show of the gladiator footwear. Brown sunglasses cover her fair face, while her short hair lays in gelled and brushed swirls on her head.

"You act like you're the one getting married," Jolene says, getting out of the car.

"The way I'm about to live vicariously through you, for a second time . . . I might as well be."

Jolene closes the door. "Girl, c'mon here. Let's hurry up and get this over with before I have to go get my kids."

"I gotta get mine too," Vaughn says. "So don't be taking too long trying on dresses and what not."

"Give me your hand," Jolene demands.

"To cross the street? We are not kids."

"Give me your hand. You know you were never good at judging traffic."

"You trippin'," Vaughn says, placing her hand in Jolene's.

The sisters run across the street hand in hand as they did when they were children. On the opposite sidewalk from where they started, they let go of each other. Jolene backs up against the outer facade of one of the boutiques and lays over her legs; her hands on her knees, head hanging down, heavy breath heaving out of her body.

"Jo, you alright?" Vaughn asks.

"I'm good. Just out of shape. I didn't say we needed to run across the street."

"If I'm holding your hand, we running," Vaughn says.

"You used to do that when we were kids, too."

"I hated holding your hand then, when Mama and Daddy would make me do it, and I for damn sure don't need to do it now. I'm grown."

"Vaughn, calm down. It was just for fun."

"So was running."

Jolene coughs once and then twice. She is still breathing heavy by the time she stands straight up. Blowing air out of her mouth to cover up how winded she is, Jolene turns around to face one of the glass shop doors, and fixes her hair. She primps and preens in the mirror, smoothing and tucking the same patches and strands of her long hair around her face, until her breath normalizes and her head stops spinning.

"So, are we going to go in the store, or are you just going to look at yourself?" Vaughn asks.

"Why are you so damn loud?" Jolene snaps.

She whips her head to glare at her sister. She has to blink rapidly to keep her vision from clouding and her head from spinning again.

"Because you're taking too damn long. I want to see you in these dresses. Hurry up."

"How you gon' be a bridezilla and you ain't never been a bride? Let's go."

"You just gotta stomp all over my dreams, don't you?" Vaughn says, following Jolene into the boutique.

"I'm not stomping all over your nothing," Jolene says. "If you wanted to be married, you could have been. Twice. You sent those rings back."

"I'm not trying to settle," Vaughn says, removing her sunglasses as she steps into One Fine Day Bridal. "I don't want to get in a marriage and then look up and want something different, and I don't even know what that something different is."

Jolene glares at Vaughn. She doesn't say anything to defend her feelings from a few weeks ago. Vaughn accepts the challenge in Jolene's eyes with one of her own, and waits for her sister to start their verbal spar. Jolene looks away and walks further into the bridal showroom. They are surrounded by dresses in every shade of white or pink, and every fabric made for opulence and elegance. Lace, satin, chiffon, and beaded, tulle dresses are crammed on the racks, lining the perimeter of the large showroom.

"Do you have an appointment?" a lilting voice calls from the back.

"No," Vaughn says, as the white woman dressed in all black, comes into view. "We're just looking."

"Well, take your time and let me know if you'd like me to pull any looks for you," the woman says addressing Vaughn.

Jolene doesn't take offense to the shop owner, writing her off. It's happened to her most of her life when she is out shopping with her sisters. The sales people always approached them, clamoring to help the thin sisters, completely ignoring the thick girl behind them.

"It's for me, actually," Jolene says.

She holds up her left hand and waves her wedding rings in the woman's face. "My husband and I are renewing our vows."

"Oh, that's wonderful," the woman says with high pitched surprise. "I'm Tricia. Feel free to look around and let me know if you need anything. Do you know what size you are?"

"I'll figure it out," Jolene says.

"Thanks, Tricia," Vaughn says.

She gives her a tight-lipped smile until she walks away. Vaughn looks at Jolene, and the two burst out laughing as they approach the racks. Jolene thumbs through the dresses still chuckling to herself.

"So, what do you want to wear?" Vaughn asks.

"Something I can fit. I don't even think I want another wedding."

"Then why'd you say yes?"

The same reason I said yes the first time.

"Because he was so sweet the way he asked. He was really excited."

"So why the change of heart?"

"Because I'd rather go on a real honeymoon than get remarried. We've already done it."

"Then tell him that. Ooh, what about this one?" Vaughn gushes.

She pulls out a white lace halter dress with see-through cleavage and a trumpet skirt. Vaughn hangs it in front of all the other dresses on that section of the rack to show off the detail. Jolene fingers the dress in her hands, and then turns it from front to back.

"It's backless," she says.

"I know," Vaughn says. "You'd be serving ass for days."

"I can't even get in that thing," Jolene says. "I can't get into any of these little ass off the rack dresses in here."

"We'll find you something," Vaughn says. "Even if you have to walk the aisle in a thong."

"I guess," Jolene says.

She walks to a corner in the showroom and sits in the lone chair in the corner and let's Vaughn pick dresses for her. She watches her sister's excitement rise with each find. It begins in her feet. Vaughn's heels start tapping on the wooden floor first, and then the movement runs up her legs and into her knees as if she's jogging in place. Jolene smiles at Vaughn and gives her a thumbs up or thumbs down to each dress. It is the only energy she can muster when her mind is twenty minutes and nearly twenty miles away, inside a hulking hospital complex that specializes in one disease. Her mind is back in the room where Doctor Richards suggested her mole may be more than a mole, more than a bump on her skin, and more than a stress pimple on a strange part of her body. Jolene's mind takes her back to the exam table where she sat staring at the mounted magazine rack that only held medical pamphlets. There were six; each of them espousing the importance of knowing the signs for diseases that can kill you. With her last look in the mirror, Jolene grabbed one of each from the Plexiglas rack before leaving the office with her file, to make a follow-up appointment. She shoved the pamphlets in her purse. They are there now sitting atop all of her other junk: wallet, keys, sunglasses, comb, brush, edge control, peppermints, butterscotch candy, day planner, phone, and a wooden fan in case she gets hot. The pamphlets for diabetes, stroke, heart disease, pregnancy, ovarian cancer, and breast cancer all sit at the top of her unzipped purse. They are the first thing she sees when she opens it. A constant reminder to what she doesn't want to be true.

Maybe Mosiah is right, Jolene thinks giving in to the one thought she's long denied. *Maybe something is wrong.*

Jolene lays her head back against the wall as Vaughn continues to pull dresses. Tricia hovers on their periphery with a watchful eye, looking over at Jolene for her approval for every dress Vaughn pulls, ready to gather them up and set up a room. Jolene ignores them both. She lays her head against the wall and closes her eyes, and waits for yet another dizzy spell to pass, and for her vision to come back into focus.

"I think this is the one, Jo," Vaughn says.

"It looks like a cloud," Jolene says.

"I think it'd be beautiful on you," Tricia says, standing closer to Vaughn.

Skinny people always want us fat girls to look bigger than we are.

"Sure, why not," Jolene says with feigned cheeriness.

This will be the easiest thing I've done all day.

Jolene stands up, pulls her waist trainer out of her purse, and then leaves the bag on the chair. She walks toward Tricia, who already has an armful of dresses. The last thing she sees before disappearing into the dressing room is Vaughn taking the seat she vacated. Her open purse is in her sister's hand. She watches as Vaughn's eyes stare at the six pamphlets inside. She looks up at Jolene.

"Right this way," Tricia says.

Jolene follows the sales woman with an armful of dresses into the curtain shrouded fitting room, ignoring the holes Vaughn bores into the back of her neck with her eyes.

Jolene's only answer is to shake her head. Her thoughts shut down the idea of any potential conversation.

Today is not the day for this. Not at all. Let's just try on these dresses and keep it cute.

12.

Wedding dress shopping was a bust. I have Vaughn to blame for that. Eight dresses, none of them remotely in a size that I could even get up past these hips, let alone my behind, and going over the top was just as useless, thanks to my arms, boobs, and back fat. I should just order a three-hundred dollar dress from China and be done with it like I did the first time around. Boutiques are overrated. And Vaughn didn't make it fun, no how, with her nosy self. Just because she saw those pamphlets in my bag doesn't mean she needed to ask me about them. All. "What's wrong with you? Jo, you okay? What was your doctor's appointment for again?" And I know she's gonna tell Tanya. Vaughn never could hold water. And Tanya's going to tell Mama, who will tell Daddy. Eventually, it will get to Granny Mae, and then she's gonna wanna lay hands on me and pour oil like she's a preacher or priestess.

This is why I hate going to the doctor in the first place. Half of their career is spent just guessing at stuff. Throw some symptoms out there and then play matchmaker with any number of diseases, not knowing which one it is. I swear, doctors and the weatherman are the only people who get to guess at their jobs and not get fired. Science my ass.

At this rate, everything in the world kills you. Food, sitting down, coffee, bacon, red meat, working . . . Everything we're used to leads to a shorter life span, and I'm supposed to lose my shit over a mole. This is Florida. Who doesn't get a suspicious mole or two? It's hot. For all Doctor Richards and Mo, know that thing could've popped up from being in the backyard one day swinging in the hammock. We may not have riverfront property like the neighbors at the end of the block, or even a house with a sewer runoff, retention pond in the back, but that doesn't mean we can't have nice accoutrements on our rectangular patch of grass. That hammock Mama and Daddy brought us back from their trip to Cancun is everything. I can lay in that thing all day.

For all Mo and Doctor Richards know, that mole could've been there two months, from laying out in the hammock in my bra on the weekends, while Lydia was napping inside, and Toussaint was either with Jemarcus or Mosiah at the shop. That's the only time I truly get to myself. Saturday during Lydia's nap when everything in my world is silent. That mole is nothing but a benign sun spot, probably, but just like everybody else in my life, Mo, overreacted. My whole life, I've been surrounded by people with a flare for the dramatic while I'm the cool, even keel girl holding everybody down, while they all act a donkey. It's the Pisces in me, just going with the flow like water. Mo, on the other hand, that Scorpio in him is always ready to strike, ready to attack a problem, even if it isn't his.

I don't know how many times I have to tell him that I'm not his passion project. I'm not his anything. He doesn't possess me. He doesn't own me. I am his wife because I want to be . . . No. Because I choose to be, because Lord knows there are some days when I don't want to be. Like the day he texted me about the appointment. That was not his problem to solve. That was not his issue to attack and take care of. It has nothing to do with him; and then of course he goes and he makes everything about him, humming those old ass songs in the process. He's the only man I know walking around humming gospel and R&B in the same breath.

I'm glad nothing is wrong with me, because I don't know what he's going to do if I'm not around. Nobody in this house can fend for themselves without me. That's why I can't stop. I can't slow down. I can't fail and still succeed. That's the cause of my stress . . . My job, my husband and family, and now this damn mole Doctor Richards says may not be a mole.

We'll see if her young ass believes her own hype. She looks like she just got out of medical school, and now she's a specialist. In what? Taking my money? That's it. High ass copay. I know the insurance better not send me no bill, talking about it's out of network, or what they don't cover.

I'm just thankful Mosiah wasn't there to ask questions. Things would be a lot different from where we are now. I'm surprised he hasn't come in here to ask me how it went yet. He wanted to do Lydia's bedtime routine tonight, since he got home early from whatever building he was cleaning. Baby, be my guest. That girl found and worked my last nerve today. She must've known I had a free day the way she carried on whining for anything, everything, throwing tantrums like she's two. Even Toussaint was more sick of her than he usually is, and I couldn't tell *him he was wrong for yelling at her, because it took everything in me not to scream right with Toussaint, "Shut up!"*

These kids. You gotta love 'em, but nobody said I had to like them all the time. Toussaint I like. Lydia, we'll see. Her little personality is hot and cold. I don't know where she got it from. Probably my mama. Mama knows she only likes being bothered when she feels like it. I'll see how long it takes her to call me about going to the doctor. See what all Vaughn said before I say anything, because I for damn sure didn't tell her nothing.

Jolene sighs to herself and drops her pen in the journal.

"Two more weeks and this will all be over," she says.

She opens the nightstand, places the journal inside, and closes it back up again. Jolene gets off the bed and walks to the bathroom, pulling off her clothes as she goes. She leaves her orange blouse, and dark wash stretchy denim and body shaper on the floor beside the tub. Pulling back the shower curtain she gets into the claw-foot tub, grabs her shower cap from the caddy, and turns on the water. Jolene waits until the water gets warm before she steps beneath the constant stream. The water beats on her covered head, and falls down her swaying body. She closes her eyes. With her arms folded beneath her breasts, she rocks from side to side. The fingers of her left hand splay in the folds of her skin, looking for what she can't ignore. The mole, the bump, the embedded red bean tucked deep in the epidermis of her body. She pulls and tugs at it, willing it to detach itself from her insides. Jolene pulls and pulls until the surrounding skin is sore.

She sways beneath the shower, leaning into the curtain. She leans too far and stumbles. Her eyes fly open, and her hands grab the air struggling to find balance. She pulls at the curtain. It flies around the ringed rod mounted to the ceiling, exposing her flailing wet body. Jolene thrusts her body forward and grabs the back of the tub. Finally steady, she flips over and sits down in the empty tub.

Jolene sighs and tries to relax again. She lays her head against the back of the tub and closes her eyes. She leaves the open shower curtain she snatched in her frenzy to regain her balance as it is. The water runs over her thighs knees and feet. Jolene scoots further down into the tub until her toes reach the opposite edge, and the steady drops of the shower are now over her belly, breasts and arms, folded beneath her chest. Hands splayed, Jolene fingers the differences in her skin texture from the right side to the left. The marked side and the unmarked side. The area raising Mosiah and Doctor Richards concerns versus the side that got little to no attention.

Laying in the tub, the shower running over her, misting gentle drops of water across her face, Jolene lets her mind wander to her family. Her mother and father in their late sixties, still in good health. Both of them still spry and energetic. Her mother runs marathons, her father cheers from the sidelines. He prefers exercise that is less strenuous. A sport that requires quiet and patience. Walking and fishing. That is his thing. That's what she shared with him, what they did together. Walking and fishing. They were bigger, but they were active. Both of them taking after her grandfather. Papa Rae. He was a big man; larger than life in both personality and size. He died right before Toussaint was born. His death almost made Granny Mae take back her promise to watch Toussaint so Jolene could finish high school. She was counting on having help, but that was snatched away by a massive heart attack. He was dead before his slumped over body hit the ground in their bedroom. That made Granny Mae start eating different. She was never a big woman, but she lost weight anyway, switching from canned vegetables to fresh ones. She started her own garden in her backyard and began walking Toussaint in his stroller around the neighborhood. Everybody in the family was health conscious, even if they couldn't afford it. Tanya and Vaughn ran with

Nikesha Elise Williams

her mother, Granny Mae walked with Toussaint, and she walked with her dad.

Granny Mae's only issue is she's old. Her body just can't do everything it used to do for long periods of time. Ain't nothing wrong with nobody else. Tanya, Vaughn, Mama, Daddy. All of them are fine. I know I don't have anything to worry about.

Jolene hears the door to the bathroom open.

"What are you doing?" Mosiah asks.

"Taking a shower," Jolene answers.

"Then why are you laying in the tub with the curtain pulled back like that." He walks over to her. "You know the floor is soaking wet."

"Sorry," Jolene says. "I fell. So I just stayed down. I'll dry the floor when I get out."

"How did you fall?" Mosiah asks, kneeling down beside her.

"I leaned too far and forgot there wasn't a back wall to catch me, and I fell."

"You okay?"

"Yeah. I'm fine."

He extends his hand. "Let me help you."

Jolene looks at Mosiah and studies his face. She sees the question he wants to ask burning behind his eyes, squinted in intensity as he assesses her body. She gives him one hand and then the other. He pulls her to her feet, but doesn't let go. He holds her hand and reaches out to the shower caddy, where he grabs one glove and the bottle of soap. He hands her both items and then holds up his free hand.

"You alright?" she asks.

"Just put the glove on my hand."

Jolene puts one glove on Mosiah's free hand and then pours the soap. She holds it up after she's done.

"Just drop it in the tub," he says.

The bottle thuds once she releases it to the ground. It rolls to the other end and clinks against the metal stopper.

"Get under the water," Mosiah says.

Jolene steps forward under the stream, still holding Mosiah's hand. He runs his gloved and soaped hand under the water to moisten the soap. Lathering it with just the tips of his fingers, he lays a flat hand on Jolene's back, holding it there until she steadies, until her breath sounds normal, and her heartbeat slows down. He lathers her back, butt, legs, and shoulders with purpose, and not provocation, with mission instead of sexual motive.

"Turn around," he says.

Jolene spins slowly. Mosiah continues soaping her body. The front of her legs, the tops of her feet, between her toes, forearms, stomach, chest, her neck. He misses nothing, leaving her femininity for last. When he's done, he holds up his hand in front of her. Jolene removes the glove and rinses beneath the shower. Mosiah lets go of her hand. He takes the one glove from her, and picks up the dropped bottle of soap from the bottom of the tub, and places both in the caddy. Turning the water off, he takes her hand and helps her step out of the tub, onto the small square bath mat that's supposed to absorb excess water. Mosiah let's her go to grab her towel. Jolene watches him move around the bathroom, sliding across the wet floor in his socks, catering to her.

I must be stupid. Any woman would happily take him from me. Hell, if I was single, I would take him from me.

Mosiah wraps Jolene in the large bath towel, and then pulls the shower cap from her head. The straight strands fall to her damp back and shoulders. Jolene gathers the ends together and tucks them to one side of her face.

"I was thinking," she says.

"About what?" Mosiah asks.

"Maybe, instead of a vow renewal next year . . ."

"Uh, huh . . ."

"Maybe we take a trip instead. Do a real honeymoon."

"Why the change of heart?"

"No change . . ."

"Are you sure?" Mosiah interrupts. "You know you tried to call off the first wedding."

"I'm sure. This isn't like that. I just think, since we never got the chance to go anywhere the first time, it might be easier this time around."

Jolene walks away from Mosiah into the bedroom. She sits on the edge of the bed, opens the nightstand, and pulls out a jar of body butter.

Laying against the closed door of the bedroom, he asks, "Can't we do both?"

Jolene scoops a hefty dose of the cream into her hand, lifts her knee to her chest, and moisturizes her skin.

She says, "I think with everything going on it may be easier to plan a trip for a year from now instead of a wedding."

"It's not a wedding, Jo. It's a vow renewal."

"Same difference. I'm still going to need a dress, we need a venue, invitations, flowers, food, a DJ. After all that, we could be on vacation. That's a lot to pick and choose and plan in ten months with everything else that's going on."

"What else is going on, Jo?"

"Nothing."

He sighs. "Since you won't just tell me, I'll ask. What did the doctor say?"

"She scheduled me for a biopsy in two weeks."

"So it's not a pimple or a mole?"

"She didn't say what it was. She just said she wanted to check it out further."

"What about the mammogram I scheduled you for?" Mosiah asks.

"We didn't do it. She just checked me out and ordered a biopsy."

"So what does that mean?"

"I don't know. I'm not the doctor."

"And of course you didn't ask."

"Mo, calm down. It's nothing. It doesn't hurt, it's not bothering me. She just wants to check to make sure."

"I told you," Mosiah said.

"Well, you better hope you're wrong because if you're right, I'm going to have a lot going on trying to plan a wedding, and dealing with whatever the hell this is. It's too much."

"I thought you said nothing was wrong," Mosiah says.

"I don't think anything is wrong. I'm just telling you what the doctor said."

"Jo, you can get the biopsy, we can plan the wedding, and we can take a honeymoon. We can do it all."

That's what got me into this marriage in the first place. Him talking about I can have it all.

He says, "I even came up with a hashtag for us."

"You've been thinking about this a lot," Jolene says.

"I have. I actually came up with two."

She smiles. "Okay, what are they?"

"The first one is easy. It's just Walker Wedding. And the second one is MoJo Getting Married. Get it," he says moving close to her. "Because I'm Mo and you're Jo, and we're getting married."

She laughs. "Yeah, I get it."

"So we're going to do it all then?" Mosiah asks, standing in front of her.

Jolene looks up at Mosiah and sees the earnest anxiety in his face. The look he only shows to her when he's putting on a front, but wants her to think he's thought of every outcome and every possibility for any number of life's situational permutations.

"Yeah, we can do it all," she says.

Mosiah leans toward Jolene until their foreheads touch and he kisses her lips. He presses his mouth to hers, imprinting himself on her body, and then pulls back.

"Let me go," Mosiah says. "I need to cut the grass."

"It's after nine," Jolene says.

"And?"

"The kids are asleep and it's dark outside."

"I'm not afraid of the dark," Mosiah says. "And you know good and well Toussaint is not sleep."

"Lydia is."

"As hard as she sleeps, she's not waking up no time soon."

"Well, how are you going to see?"

"I can see, and we have a light on the patio. I'll be fine."

"Why can't you just wait until the weekend?"

"Because it's been bothering me for days. I told Toussaint to do it, and he never did."

"I didn't know you wanted him to cut the grass. Why didn't you tell me?"

"Because I told *him*. That's alright. He's mine on Saturday. Might as well tell Jemarcus now. Not this weekend."

"Fine by me," Jolene says.

She pulls down the towel to rub the butter cream into her upper body.

"See now you playing," Mosiah says.

"What? I'm putting on lotion."

"And, I'm going to cut the grass."

Mosiah opens and closes the door, leaving Jolene in the room. He walks the hallway, peeking in on Toussaint, laying spread eagle across the bed, and then looks in on Lydia, snuggled up beneath her own covers. Mosiah races down the stairs and out to the garage to start up the lawnmower, hoping the steady roar of the cutting engine will drown the thoughts running through his mind; her voice saying the word "biopsy" in the incessant refrain of some tortuous military tactic.

13.

Biopsy.
I guess some things are better left unsaid.
Mosiah pushes the lawnmower in a rectangular pattern across the backyard for a second time. The smell of gas and grass permeate his nose, creating a noxious scent he should have abandoned to an hour ago, when he finished the yard the first time. He's purposefully shredding the grass, cutting it down nearly to its root, to keep from going back inside. To keep from facing Jolene. To keep from putting on a brave front to match her own. He cuts around a lemon tree, and then the last row of grass along the fence line. Mosiah finally cuts the engine when he butts up against the fence, in the final corner of their property.
Biopsy.
She said biopsy. I thought it was just a cyst they were going to have to drain or something. I don't know what I thought. Not this.
The song changes in Mosiah's headphones as he pushes the lawnmower across the grass to the open garage. A soulful scale of piano keys blasts in his ear as he pushes the lawnmower back in its place in the garage. His pickup truck is parked next to her SUV, and there's still room enough in the garage for everything they have shoved in corners, stacked on shelves, and hanging from nails. Mosiah pulls down the Weedwhacker as the tortured voice of a seventies soul singer tells him about the many places he's been in his lifetime. He walks to the front of the house and turns on the motor for the machine to edge the grass that's been cut too low.

His mind is on his heart that lives outside of his body, beating in the body of the woman, in the upstairs bedroom. Her face comes into focus as the song tells of loving in a place where there's no space or time. He sees her in all of her variations: when they were toddlers, children, adolescents, teenagers, adults, husband and wife, and now parents. He remembers the changing shape of her face with every phase. Whether her cheeks were chubby from excess weight or angular from losing too much, she was always the same inside. The woman he claimed as his wife before he knew that's what he wanted, the girl he made sure fell asleep before him, the wife whose son he loved as his own because they both loved her.

Mosiah edges the last side of the front yard until the dirt demarcation is so deep, the gulch so crisp that the remnants of the tattered grass look like they're floating beneath the moonlight. He walks to the garage as the song changes. The whining of an organ comes through the headphones, followed by a succession of chords, before another tenor voice assaults his aural atmosphere. Mosiah hangs up the Weedwhacker on a nail and closes the garage door as the voice sings out his good days and bad days. In the pitch black darkness of the space, filled with the things for a life lived outside, Mosiah sings along with the familiar gospel song. He belts the song usually only sung at funerals to comfort the grieving and remind the mourning, death is also apart of God's plan.

Mosiah sings through the air that holds the thick scent of gasoline, grass, and his own sweat. He sings into the space he's occupying as his cavern, his man cave, the room for his emotions. No one can see him with sweat dripping from his body and tears rolling from his eyes. Toussaint, Lydia, and Jolene are asleep above him in their bedrooms. The neighbors are mostly asleep in the homes beside him. In the darkness of the night, inside the tar hollow of his creation, Mosiah pours out his building frustration as the song comes to the climax about drying tears away and turning midnights into day.

Out of breath, Mosiah's voice cracks with contravention as his body won't allow his mouth to sing what he does not yet believe. He inhales and exhales for air, but little comes. Mosiah opens the door that leads into the living area of the home. The cool air from the inside of the house fills his lungs. He closes the garage door behind him and leans against it. Looking around the room only slightly illuminated from the stove light, as the air dries the sweat on his skin, he notices the pictures hung on the walls, lining both sides of the stairwell. Their black and white wedding pictures. He focuses on Jolene in a dress he could barely get her out of from all of the tulle and tutu slips she had on beneath it. He looks from her to his seven-year younger self in a simple black suit and over polished shoes to hide the scuff marks. Beside the wedding photos are pictures of Toussaint and Lydia. They're lined up along the staircase wall that ascends to the second floor. Their baby pictures, one in black and white, and one in sepia are split by a wooden sign that says "Lord bless this house," a wedding gift from his father. Mosiah shivers in his jumpsuit. He shakes his head as he kicks off his work boots, and then picks them up. If he doesn't carry them across the room to leave on the rack by the front door, he knows Jolene will have a fit in the morning. *You left those dirty, muddy, hairy boots on my floor, and you know I just mopped.* He laughs to himself, hearing her high-pitched outrage. It is the first noticeable lift to his spirit since she said she was scheduled for a biopsy. His memory of her does more good for him than all of the music he blasted while he was outside.

With an outward smile on his face, Mosiah picks up his boots and walks them across the living room to the shoe rack at the front door. He goes upstairs, peeking in on Toussaint and Lydia again, before walking into his own bedroom.

"Jo, you awake?" he asks, softly closing the door behind him.

"How can anybody sleep with the lawnmower going and you giving a full concert in the garage like you're one of the Winans' brothers."

"Sorry. I didn't think you could hear me."

"It's not sound proof, Mo."

"Sorry, I just had a lot on my mind."

"I know. That's when you sing the loudest."

"At least I can sing."

"That's why I didn't complain. Now let me sleep."

Mosiah moves quickly across the bedroom to the closet and then the bathroom, closing doors behind him as he tries to shield Jolene from his noise. He strips out of his clothes, turns the knob to the shower, and gets into the water. Staring down at the bottom of the tub, he sees the brown dirt of outside wash away from his hair, his face, and his goatee. Flecks of grass also wash away from him as the water warms, and rains down his body.

He pours the multi-purpose soap into his hair and over his skin before grabbing the gloves. With his eyes closed tight, he scrubs from the top of his head, over his face, and down his body until the soap begins to sting. Mosiah stands steady beneath the showerhead, until all the suds are rinsed away and his body is again soaked in water.

"Another day down the drain," he says.

Mosiah turns off the shower, pulls back the curtain, and walks naked, dripping water into the bedroom.

"Jo, you sleep?" he asks.

"No," she says. "I can't."

"Sorry," he says.

Mosiah pulls back the covers and gets into the bed beside her. He throws one arm out to her waist and gathers her to him.

"Why are you naked?" Jolene asks.

"Because tonight we're sleeping naked."

"We?"

"Yes, we."

Mosiah pulls Jolene's night sweats and crop top off of her body, and throws them to the floor. He leaves her floral satin scarf in place around her head, as he buries his nose into her neck.

"What's gotten into you?" she asks.

"Nothing. Just thinking, that's all."

"About what?"

"Nothing important. It can wait."

"Must be something, it's got you singing "I Won't Complain" at the top of your lungs."

"It's nothing."

"Mo," Jolene says, turning over in his arms to face him.

"Yes, Baby."

"Why didn't you ever try to do music when you came back home?"

"Most women roll their eyes and write a brotha off if he's over twenty, talking about trying to make his music career take off."

"That's because most of those brotha's think they got bars, and they barely have a vocabulary big enough to string together a decent rhyme."

"Exactly my point?"

"But you're not rapping, Mo. You can actually sing."

"I know that, and you know that, and Lydia and TeeTee know that . . ."

"Okay, and . . ."

"And that's good enough for me. I only sing when I need to. When I don't have the words or the thoughts, I've always got a song."

"I guess I have your mother to thank for that."

"You do."

Mosiah yawns into Jolene's skin and wraps his arms around her. He says into her ear, "I love you."

"I love you too," Jolene says.

She kisses his lips and turns back over in his arms. Her bare back to his bare chest, one hand supports her head on the pillow they share, while the other holds his from the arm wrapped around her body. She closes her eyes to sleep, but her mind is wired and alert. She waits for consciousness to wane, for the nighttime functions of her subconscious to take over, for her body to transcend into the moments that she won't remember.

It eludes her. Instead, a song of her own comes to her lips. She hums the sweet melody that was accompanied by an acoustic guitar and a British voice. Mosiah picks up the harmony and adds another layer to the mood she created. Jolene opens her eyes and stares across the dark room toward the large mirror in the corner by the windows. She can't see their faces, only their forms. Their legs and bodies, one massive amorphous clump, unmoving on Mosiah's side of the bed.

He won't tell me what's wrong, and now I'm not going to get any sleep. I guess this is how he feels when I get into one of my moods.

Jolene lets the song fizzle as she brings his hand from around her body to her mouth. She kisses his knuckles and then his fingertip, before rolling over in his arms to face him again.

"You sleep?" she asks in a whisper.

Mosiah shakes his head no. Jolene kisses his nose and then his mouth. She explores the possibilities of his lips and the capabilities of his tongue, as if it was their first kiss all over again. She takes her time in the moment as if they are once again twenty-three, sneaking around her parents' house, making sure not to wake up Toussaint or her sisters. She plays in his face, rubbing her fingers across his eyebrows and down his cheeks, as she kisses the breath away from him. She smothers him with her mouth until she feels hardening growth against her softness.

Her hands move from his face, down his neck, over his collarbone, across his chest and to his lingam lingering between them. Jolene creates a trail of kisses following the same path her hands took, until her mouth works in tandem with her hands, providing warmth and pleasure to push away the thoughts he won't divulge. She buries herself in him, secreting saliva to pull the lust from his body to alleviate the anxiety in his mind. Jolene works her hands and her mouth, until she feels the texture of his contentment begin to bubble on the ridges of her lips. She devours him over and over, her head bobbing with skill until her jaws swell and pop from him pulling her to his base.

With one grip, he lifts her astride him and gives in to her wishes. He gives her the power of his body since they both know he won't reveal his thoughts. It is how they've always communicated when he was the one at the center of the inquisition. She rides him to make him relate the one way he knows how. In action, in deed, in doing something to feel useful and purposed. It is his way to comfort, to process, strategize and learn. The Scorpio in him ruling the entire exchange. The Pisces in her guiding him to release his brooding, even if it is only through his body. The water of their signs flows through both of them, deepening their emotional maturity expressed in the physicality of their interconnection.

Jolene rides Mosiah on the languid melody of the song they hummed. She strums his body with the inside of her own, discarding the occasional dissatisfaction that overcomes her, the sweeping doubt that threatens to strangle her, and the insecurity that hovers on her periphery with the intent to choke every good thing away from her. She chokes her complaints and works to pull plenary passion from their congress, until he is completely depleted and ready for discourse. This is their most intimate and innate communication.

Mosiah rolls Jolene to her back and slams into her body with the last stroke of his physical pen. He writes his uncertainties, anxieties, concerns, and questions in a place she cannot see. He buries his secrets, knowing she is the only one who will be able to find them and unlock the answers. Mosiah collapses on her still writhing body, waiting until her own mysteries have been given to him in the melisma of her waning moans. Congressed and conversed, their euphonic chorus was the necessary conversation.

Mosiah's hands feel along the length of her body, still holding her close as they separate and part. His fingers graze the anomalous growth that brought them together. The aberration that forced her to pour her thoughts in her journal, and him to exert his energy in the yard. He fingers the imposition that's triggered their dispositions. The pimple, the embodied red bean, the bump, the lump that could lead to a drastically different life. One that almost didn't happen if he had not persisted that she become his wife.

14.

"So we can still be friends, right?" Jolene asked into the cell phone receiver, pressed close against her face.

She listened intently for an answer but didn't hear one. There was only silence on the other end of the phone. She pulled it away from her ear to look at the screen and saw it was dead. The line was cleared the call was over. She sat down on her twin bed beside where Toussaint slept, and rubbed his back.

"It's just me and you now," she said, making circles across his pajama shirt. "It's just me and you now."

It's always going to be just me and you.

She sighed to herself as she laid on her back. Jolene stared at the ceiling. She stared at the bare purple walls of the room she shared with Vaughn. She glanced at Toussaint sleeping beside her, and then over at Jovon sleeping on Vaughn's bed. She made a round robin with her eyes over and over in the room, until the glancing made her dizzy and she had to close her eyes to shake the whirlwind of her glaze.

Inside her own mind, their faces came to her. Mosiah and Jemarcus. The fiancé she had just let go and the father of her son she didn't want. Jolene opened her eyes and brought her hands to her face. Slowly, she slid off the diamond engagement ring. The two carat stone in a white gold band, got stuck around her knuckle. It protested it's removal as she tried to make what she thought was the right decision permanent.

"What you doing in here with the doors closed and the lights on?" Vaughn asked, bursting into the room.

"Nothing," Jolene answered.

"Well, you could at least leave the lights off so the boys don't wake up in all this bright you got going on in here."

"Turn off the lights, Vaughn. I'll turn on the lamp."

Vaughn flipped the switch to kill the bright overhead lights in their room as Jolene turned on the lamp sitting on the floor between her be and the wall. She set the ring she was able to wedge off of her finger beside it and laid back down on the bed. Vaughn sat down beside Jovon's sleeping body, with a book and two notebooks. She kicked off one shoe and then the other, letting them flop on the floor.

"What's wrong with you?" She asked.

"I just told you nothing," Jolene snapped.

"Then if it's nothing, why aren't you wearing your ring? You can't just leave that thing sitting anywhere. You know people steal."

"You mean you steal."

"I didn't say me."

"Well, you're the only one in here and you're the only one who knows I've taken it off. Well, you and Mo."

"So why'd you take it off?" Vaughn asked.

"Because Mo and I aren't getting married."

"What do you mean, y'all not getting married? He proposed. You said yes. You've been walking around here glowing like you pregnant, even though you not knocked up. You not pregnant, are you?"

"No, Vaughn."

"So explain to me how you go from glowing to gloomy?"

"It's complicated," Jolene said, sitting up on the bed.

"Why do I have a feeling this has something to do with Jemarcus."

Jolene didn't answer. She didn't even turn her head to meet Vaughn's accusatory gaze. She reached her arms behind her back and beneath her shirt, and unclasped her bra. She pulled the straps down out of the short sleeves of her purple graphic T-shirt, and tossed it in the corner with a pile of other dirty clothes that needed to be washed.

"Because it does," Vaughn said. "What did Mr. I Like to Ruin Everybody's Lives say to you now that made you lose the last bit of good sense you had?"

Jolene looked at Vaughn; her sister who was self-righteous even in her own mistakes, and so self-assured there was never any room for doubt. She looked at Vaughn, back down to her normal size after Jovon, even though she was still struggling to lose the weight from having Toussaint. Vaughn, with her short Kelis inspired hair cut, long legs, flawless fair skin, and knowing eyes excoriated Jolene with just her gaze. Even though they were both single, teen mothers, Jolene saw the look of "I'm better than you" in her sister because of her own tendency to self-destruct.

"What happened, Jo?" Vaughn demanded.

"I called off the wedding," Jolene blurted.

"Why?"

"Because it's never going to work. Me and Mosiah. Mosiah and me, we're never going to work."

"And who told you that? Jemarcus? Because if there's anyone it's not going to work with it's him."

"No, it's not Jemarcus. I don't want him. I barely had him when I did, and he's got shit characteristics, so I know I for damn sure don't want him now."

"So why'd you dump Mo?"

"Because Mosiah was the rebound. It wasn't supposed to last. He was just something to help while I got my mind right."

"I don't believe you. I don't even think you believe you."

"Whatever," Jolene said, laying back down on the bed.

She closed her eyes and, once again, saw both men dueling for her attention, while neither one of them vied for her affection.

Marry him if you want to.

You'll never be happy.

She heard Jemarcus' bold statement loud and clear in her head. His declaration over her future he made earlier in the afternoon, when she picked up Toussaint from him.

She knocked on the door of his parents' house in the Hidden Hills subdivision, one hand on her hip, the other suspended in mid-air, ready to rap again when he flung the door open with Toussaint in one arm.

"Why isn't he dressed, Jemarcus? I told you I was on my way."

"He's got on a shirt. I was just about to put his pants on. Stop tripping."

"I'm not tripping. I just got stuff to do. You said he would be ready."

"He is. We just finished eating. Chill out. Let me put some pants on him and he's all yours," Jemarcus said. "Ain't that right lil' man."

"Yup, yup," Toussaint said in his toddler squeak.

"Hurry up." Jolene said.

"It's not gon' take but a second."

"So go!"

"You just gon' stand on the porch and wait, or are you coming inside?"

"I'm good right here," Jolene said. She folded her arms across her chest and leaned against the front door frame of the house.

"Suit yourself," Jemarcus said.

He closed the door and left Jolene to sulk against the door as she waited. She pulled her sunglasses down from where they rested on top of her hair, and shrouded her eyes from the glow of the setting sun. She drummed her fingers on her arms and elbow, waiting for Jemarcus to bring Toussaint to her. She tried not to show her irritation, keeping the agitated rock in her body to a minimum, but it was useless. What her body showed only minimally, her thoughts expounded on exponentially.

After four years of "I'm too busy. I can't make it. You need to come get him." Now all of a sudden he's got time to play dear old doting dad, like I don't have things to do. Same old Jemarcus. He only wants to be bothered when he feels like being bothered.

And I fall for it every single time.

"Go on to your mama now," Jemarcus said as he opened the door.

"Mommy, Mommy Mommy," Toussaint squealed, leaping on Jolene with open arms.

"Yes, Baby," she said, catching him.

"Me and my daddy going on an airplane."

"You are?"

"Yup, yup."

"It's yes."

"Yes."

"Where are you going?"

"Nor Car-lina,"Toussaint said.

Jolene stared at Jemarcus, waiting for him to answer her unasked question. He shrugged as she adjusted Toussaint to her other hip.

"Where's his bag?" she asked.

"Right here," Jemarcus said.

He handed her the bag letting his fingers graze hers long enough, until she looked at him and snatched her hand away.

"So what's in North Carolina that you need to take Toussaint?"

"You know that's where I'm from," Jemarcus said. "My mom and pops want to go up there in a few months for a family reunion, and they said it'd be nice if Toussaint was there with us to get to know his family."

"So now your parents want to be bothered with my baby?"

"Jolene, you need to let that go."

"I will not."

"We were kids. They were just trying to look out for my future."

"By saying they'd pay for my abortion. And then when I didn't have one, forcing you to get a DNA test, and then, still not wanting you to come around your son after it was proven he was yours. Naw, I'm not forgetting shit."

"Mommy, you owe me a quarter."

"Okay, Toussaint. I'll give it to you when we get in the car."

"Jolene, what happened happened. Now can we just move on?" Jemarcus said.

She eyed him up and down in the door frame as she held on to Toussaint and his overnight bag. She heard Doctor Fisher loud and clear in her head saying, "choose joy" as she counted backwards from ten, studying the man she used to love when he was a boy and she was a girl. In a plain white T-shirt with a chocolate stain in the center, red basketball shorts, and black sports slides, Jolene looked at Jemarcus and tried to remember what she loved about him. The sleepy eyes, the half grin, his thick Geechee drawl, she tried to remember what it was that made her lock on to him at thirteen and refuse to let go for years.

"I see you're moving on," Jemarcus said, nodding toward her left hand.

Jolene looked down at the new ring sparkling on her finger. "It's nothing," she said, hiding her hand under Toussaint's body.

"That's not what Toussaint said," Jemarcus said. "He said, 'My mommy is getting married to Mr. Mo and he's going to be my new daddy.'"

"What can I say, Jemarcus? Time moves forward."

"I'm not saying anything about it. Good on you. Mosiah finally got what he wanted."

"What the hell is that supposed to mean."

"Mommy, you owe me two quarters," Toussaint said.

"Mommy will give you a dollar when we get in the car," Jolene said.

Jemarucs continued, "Mo was always jealous when we were together. I guess he finally wore you down. It takes a special kind of man to know he's not wanted and still go after what he can't have."

"You're so fucked up."

"Three quarters," Toussaint said.

"I told you I was going to give you a dollar. That's the same as four quarters, Baby. Now be quiet. Mommy's talking to your dumb ass daddy."

"Oh, so now I'm a dumb ass?" Jemarcus asked.

"You are, when you assume I can't be happy with someone who actually loves me, and treats me right. Oh, I must only be with him because I can't have you. Get the fuck over yourself, Jemarcus. You are nobody's prize. You ain't even doing shit with your life."

"That's why I hate getting him," Jemarcus said. "Everytime I see you, I see all my mistakes, and you just love to rub that shit in."

"Then go back to not seeing him like you been doing. You just asked for him so you could talk to me about Mo. That's not your business. If it's not about Toussaint, you don't get to talk to me about it."

"Ain't nobody studyin' you and Mosiah. Church boy ain't got shit on me. Marry him if you want to. If you think that will make you feel better, because I didn't want your fat ass. You'll never be happy."

"Fuck you, Jemarcus. Fuck you."

Jolene stormed off away from the door jostling Toussaint from side to side. She strapped him in quickly to his booster seat, got in the car, and sped away as quickly as she could from his door. She drove out of the subdivision named for the golf course that was built inside of it, and drove back to her parents' home, his words echoing the entire way.

Marry him if you want to.
You'll never be happy.

The words she didn't want to affect her did, as she sat in her room beside Toussaint staring from her ring to her phone, trying to decide if marriage would make her happy, or if she'd rather just be single.

I never even thought about marriage.

Mosiah deserves better than this. Better than me. Better than somebody else's sloppy seconds.

Jolene's own thoughts drove her to make the phone call. To call off the wedding. To suggest just being friends, as they had always been. But Mosiah's non-agreement didn't sit right with her. He didn't say okay, he didn't say goodbye, the line clicked and she was left in the room with her son and her thoughts. A ring she should have rejected and a sister who didn't understand.

Jolene opened her eyes. Vaughn was still there. Still staring at her, her big eyes asking what happened.

"Stop looking at me like that," Jolene said, sitting back up on the bed.

"Not until you tell me why you tossed aside a perfectly good man who adores you, over an idiot."

"Jemarcus is not an idiot," Jolene defends.

"Then you're the idiot for saying that."

"Vaughn, you don't understand."

"Then make me understand," Vaughn said, crossing from her bed to Jolene's bed.

"I want to be married but not like this. Mo is getting over stuff from the war, I'm getting right from Jemarcus. Hurt recognizes hurt. We're just using each other, and now I see it for what it is."

"And what's that?"

"Somebody to help me to move on to who I'm really supposed to be with."

"And who is that?" Vaughn asked.

"Myself," Jolene answered assuredly. "Right now I think I'm supposed to be by myself."

Vaughn wrapped her arms around Jolene, unsure of what she could say that would be received, to make her big sister see herself and her life differently. Side by side on the twin bed, they rocked back and forth as Vaughn tried to create a comfort Jolene still couldn't feel. In her bare arms, she tried to impart, and infuse her own feelings she felt into her sister's spirit. Beauty and bodaciousness, courage and fearlessness, grit and determination, strength and humility. Vaughn rocked with Jolene on the bed until Jolene heaved a sigh, breaking free from the embrace.

She said, "Mo is better off without me. He's better off finding a girl that will really make him happy, instead of someone with all this baggage. I'm still trying to figure myself out. How can I be somebody's wife?"

"If you really believe that, then fine. But if that's some Jemarcus reverse psychology, I don't want you and I don't want nobody else to want you bullshit, then you need to stop letting him get in your head and get back what you really want before it's too late."

"But I'm not sure I even want Mo."

"You said yes."

"Only after I ran out of excuses to say no. Do you know how many times I tried to get him to standup without putting that ring on my finger. Why do you think we took so long to rejoin the party?"

"I thought y'all were confessing your love to one another. I don't know."

"No. I was trying to get him to call it off before it even began."

"Why?" Vaughn asked as she reached over to hold Jolene's hand.

"Because he's too good for me."

"Who told you that?"

"No one. It's just true."

"Jolene, why don't you think you deserve to win? That you deserve to be happy?"

"I didn't say that."

"Maybe not those exact words, but you said it. Why are you letting Jemarcus get in your head and ruin everything you and Mosiah have going?"

"And what do me and Mo have? Huh? What do we have?"

"You've known each other forever, he came to the hospital when Toussaint was born, you wrote him while he was all over the world in the military."

"And then he came home and didn't even tell me he was back. He ghosted me just like Jemarcus."

"He lost a friend in the service, JoJo. He was hurt. But you found him anyway and y'all picked up wherever the letters left off."

Jolene sighed. She heard the reason, but didn't feel swayed to pick up the phone and undo what she had already done. She looked from where her sister held her hand to the ring she left sitting by the lamp to Toussaint's sleeping body on the bed beside her. She started her ocular gymnastics all over again, beating her lashes rapidly against her lower lids to blink back the tears that threatened to well up. She tried to shutter with her own eyes the emotion she stuffed inside, until her pain felt so numb she didn't know it was there.

Jolene collapsed on the bed. She let her body fall away from Vaughn as she brought her naked fingers to her face to hide the tears she could no longer refuse to cry. Vaughn sat beside her watching, stroking the top of her leg. She sat in the sniffling, snuffing heart cry of her sister's melancholy remorse, staring across the bed at her own son. Her own toddler begotten before heartache, wanting to cry her own tears but unable to compel them to roll down her face. Vaughn sat beside Jolene, letting her express what they both felt for different reasons. Jolene who had let go of both what she wanted and didn't want because of self-doubt, cried into her pillow and Toussaint's shoulder, letting her body perseverate with the flood of her own hapless thoughts. Vaughn sat beside her, holding her own news to herself, her own source of pride and contention.

As Jolene cried she lifted up her sea green tank top and looked at her belly. She looked at the line that proved she bore Jovon, and wondered how dark it would get with the new life no one else knew was inside of her. The life created during an impromptu make up, that didn't last a day. Vaughn squeezed the sides of her body, folded the skin of her belly in on itself, and wondered how long it would take this time, before she started showing. She looked at her navel innately tucked in it's own cavern and wondered how long it would take to pop forward with the rounded bigness of a head, shoulders, arms, hands, legs and feet.

Vaughn stood up from the bed and walked back to her own and sat down beside Jovon. She said, "I don't know what Jemarcus said to you, JoJo, and I don't know what you and Mosiah's relationship is like. But if you're letting one influence the other, it sounds to me like he doesn't want you to be happy, and you're allowing him to make that decision for you."

Jolene didn't respond in the moment. It was interrupted by a rapping at their window. Jolene's bed was directly beneath it. She sat up in the bed and looked out to see Mosiah's face staring back at her tearstained cheeks.

"He's bold," Vaughn said.

"Open the window, Jolene," Mosiah demanded from outside.

"What are you doing here?"

"I came to see you."

His words reach her in a warble, due to the thick glass and wood between them. She presses her face close to the window to make sure he can see her lips as she speaks. In a voice just above a whisper, she says, "Now you see me. Go home, Mo."

"No. You're just as fucked up about this as I am."

"I'll be fine, Mo," Jolene said.

"Come outside."

"No."

Jolene laid back down on the bed beneath the window, not caring that Mosiah could look in and see her. She wiped her eyes, even though her pillow was still wet with the residue from where she poured out her feelings. Vaughn looked from Jolene to Mosiah and back again. Mosiah stared at them through the window and mouthed, "Help me."

"So you're just going to lay here in the bed crying, when the man has literally driven all the way over here, even though you just rejected him and turned down his proposal," Vaughn said.

"I didn't tell him to come over here."

"Exactly. He's here on his own. If that's not love, JoJo, I don't know what is."

"We're friends."

"Then if y'all are real friends go outside and talk to him."

"For what, Vaughn? For what?"

"Because friends face each other even when shit has gone to hell in a hand basket."

"Fine," Jolene said, popping up off the bed. "I'm coming," she yelled toward the window. "Vaughn, watch Toussaint."

"Don't I always?"

Vaughn laid down on her own bed, next to Jovon, with her hands beneath her belly, longing to feel the kick of love that was waiting for Jolene outside their window.

Outside, Jolene could hear the crickets and the frogs singing their nightly song as she walked to the back of the house to where her bedroom was and where Mosiah waited. In pink furry house shoes, jeans, a T-shirt, and no bra, she approached Mosiah with her hands over her breasts to hold them down. In the dim light of the moon, she saw he looked as distraught as she felt. His face was ashen; his T-shirt and shorts wrinkled.

She said, "I'm here."

"I see," Mosiah said. "I see you took off your ring."

Jolene tucked her hands so her left wouldn't show. "What do you want?" she asked.

"I want you to say it to my face."

"Say what?"

"You want to call off the wedding. You don't want to be with me. You want to just be friends. Say it to my face."

"I want to just be friends," Jolene blurted, looking down at the patch of grass they stood in.

"Look me in my eye and say it. Come over here," he pointed, "and say it to my face."

"Mo, I just said it. I said it on the phone. I said it when you proposed. This isn't going to work. I'm not what you need. Let's just be friends."

"How can you tell me what I need?"

"I can't, but whatever it is you do need, I know that I'm not it."

"Jolene, that's the furthest thing from the truth."

"You'll find somebody else," she insisted.

Mosiah sighed. He closed the gap between them and invaded her space. He stood in front of her toe to toe; nearly navel to navel and nose to nose. He longed to reach out and grab her; a hand, her hip, but he kept himself to himself until she invited him closer. He wanted her to want him as much as he wanted her, to need him as much as he needed her. He wanted what he felt to be reciprocated instead of shunned. He wanted her to know that even though at one point he shut her out, her letters, all the old ones he'd read and the few she sent after his silence, kept him from taking his own gun, and putting it in his mouth to ease the guilt and grief he felt for losing the man who fought beside him. He wanted to tell her how she kept him alive when he didn't feel fit to live, when survivor's remorse drowned him, and he could no longer see the flash of his gun going off into enemies of war he was trained to kill.

"Don't do this, JoJo," Mosiah said.

"I'm not doing anything."

"Yes, you are."

"Mo, why do you want to be with me? Tell me why you want to marry me? Tell me why you want me to be your wife? Tell me why me, when you could have a million girls throwing you ass any day of the week?"

"Because it's not about the ass, the sex, the looks, the shape. That doesn't do shit for me. It's about the person. The spirit. The soul. The connection. Mine has always connected with yours. You know that."

"There's no such thing as preschool sweethearts, Mo."

"Maybe not, but we ain't in preschool and I still love you. It's always been you, JoJo, and you know it."

Jolene sighed. She let the tears she cried inside, spill out in front of him.

Why do you keep doing this?

She questioned herself. She questioned him. With her arms folded, her eyes flowing, and her thoughts running, she stood in front of Mosiah, letting him see all that he was asking for. She didn't wipe her tears, or move the hair that stuck to her face and began to shrivel with the water her own body produced.

"You should go," she said.

"Nah, I'm good," Mosiah said, bending down to the ground.

He sat on the grass and leaned his head against the brick facade of the home beneath Jolene's window. One leg extended in front of him, and one knee pulled into his chest, he crossed his arms over his body, closed his eyes and began to hum. She'd heard him humming before, but rarely anything she recognized. This time she could hear the pain and sadness in the gospel tune sung in times of hardship, or in times of rejoicing when hardship ended.

"I'm going inside," Jolene said.

"I'll be here," Mosiah said.

"Mo, you can't stay out here all night. You should go home and get some sleep."

"If I get tired I'll sleep right here."

"You can't sleep outside, Mo."

"It's not like it's the first time. I'm good, JoJo. Get some sleep. I'll be here."

Jolene started to protest but decided against it. She turned around in the grass and walked to the front of the house, went inside, and back to her bedroom. She returned to a darkened room where she had to feel her way through, to not to wake up Vaughn or their boys. By memory and touch she found her bed. She pushed Toussaint closer to the wall beneath the window and crawled in close on her side. Her head on the pillow, eyes closed, tears yet a trickle, she heard him. The deep hum, and then the growl as good days and bad days poured out of Mosiah, singing her soul to sleep.

"I didn't know he could sing," Vaughn said through the darkness.

"Yeah, he can," Jolene said.

"Why is he out there?"

"Because he didn't leave."

"And you're just going to let him stay out there?"

"Yeah. I'm tired. I can't do this with him tonight."

"Well then, I guess y'all will do it in the morning because it doesn't seem like he's going to leave no time soon."

"He'll leave," Jolene assured.

"And if he doesn't?" Vaughn asked.

"Then I'll see him in the morning."

"You mean Mama will see him in the morning."

"She may. It doesn't matter."

Nothing matters.

Jolene fell asleep to Mosiah singing "I Won't Complain" over and over. It was the first time she heard the song from his lips, that she would later learn, was his go to whenever he was feeling a kind of way. By the time she awoke the next morning, the tenor outside her window was silent. The bed across from her was empty, and the sun was high and burning. She looked at the time on the old alarm clock beside the lamp on the floor, and saw it was an hour after she normally dropped Toussaint off at daycare. Jolene rushed around the room to get him ready and get him dressed, and then herself.

"Mommy, your ring," Toussaint said to her as she ushered him out of the room.

"I don't need it, Baby," she said.

"But Mr. Mo said you were never gonna take it off. Put it back on."

"I don't need it, Baby," Jolene said again.

"C'mon Mommy, put it on. Mr. Mo said."

"Give it to me, Toussaint.

He quickly swiped the ring from the floor and hurried it over to Jolene. She shoved it on her finger and then carried him out of the house. In the driveway, Mosiah's pickup truck was still there beside her old Camry. She pulled Toussaint around to the back side of the house and saw that he was still there, beneath her window, one leg extended, the other drawn to him, head leaned against the bricks with his eyes closed.

"Mommy, why is Mr. Mo sleeping outside?" Toussaint asked.

"I don't know." Jolene answered.

"Can I ask him?"

"I'm not sleeping, TeeTee. I'm just waiting."

"How long have you been up waiting?" Jolene asked.

"Since your mom sprayed me with the sprinklers this morning."

"Sorry about that," Jolene said, trying to conceal her smirk. "I didn't think you'd really be out here all night."

"You still haven't told me why you don't want to do this. Why we should "just be friends" as you say."

"And you still haven't said why you're so pressed for me to be your wife. So I guess we're even."

"I see you put your ring back on," Mosiah said, nodding at her finger.

"Toussaint made me put it back on."

"He's four."

"He's the boss."

"Well, I'm glad you put it back on," Mosiah said.

"You didn't give me much choice about it either," she said.

"Jolene, you always have a choice. You just need to have an explanation behind your choices."

"I know."

"Then I'm glad you made the right one."

"I have to get Toussaint to school," Jolene said.

"I get it. I'll go," Mosiah said, standing up.

He walked over toward her and then the three of them walked together to their cars. He didn't mention he spoke to her mother after he got sprayed with the water from the sprinklers. He didn't tell her that her mother told him to be patient, and that she'd come around. He didn't voice his own fear that she may not and he'd be out a lover and a friend. He walked her to her car, helped her tuck Toussaint into his seat, and then cornered her when she closed the door. Toe to toe, nearly navel to navel and nose to nose, he looked deep into her freshly washed face, sans makeup and memorized the visage of her vulnerability.

He said, "If you really don't want to do this, tell me why and I'll go."

In the light of the new day, Mosiah's insistent eyes beaming down on her, and his worn complexion staring back at her, she didn't repeat her aphoristic maxims or pessimistic platitudes she barely believed herself. She nodded, leaned up toward his face, and planted a simple kiss on his dry lips. She pressed away her fears and insecurities, Jemarcus' words, and Mosiah's own troubles. He pressed back against her lips coated with gloss to seal their deal.

He said, "I want you to be my wife because I like the way I feel when I'm around you. Your words make my days easier, and your love makes my nights less lonely. I want that everyday. I want you everyday."

"Okay," Jolene said.

She stopped trying to push away what she knew she needed, what she really wanted despite her own doubts, not knowing the same restlessness would show up again, years later, a baby later, when she would be forced to decide if having each other was enough, at a time when he became all she had.

15.

I've had an annual, an ultrasound, an MRI, and a biopsy, and they still don't know what this is. They still haven't told me if I'm free to go back to living my life before this interruption of everything, by something they can't even name.

Jolene's mind races over the thoughts she poured into her journal before coming into the doctor's office. Her uncertainties, her worries, her anxiety grew with every stroke of her pen. The curves and the lines of every word she formed, stoked her fears instead of expurgating them out of her body and into the book, where she loosed her conscience in the name of internal stability.

She sits in the office, fully clothed waiting for the doctor. This visit is different from the last two she's had. Then, they asked their perfunctory questions about how she felt, and took her vitals, and that was all. Now they've shoved her in a room and are making her wait. They are making both of them wait.

Mosiah sits across from Jolene in the chair behind the undrawn curtain. His expression is pensive. Hands steepled in front of his nose, worry lines etched in his face, she sees his feelings beyond his facade. He was alert, determined, and attentive when she told him yesterday that she had to come into the office today for her results; that they couldn't give them to her over the phone.

He said, "I'm coming with you."

It was not a question and he did not ask permission. It was a statement of fact, his truth; that no matter what appointments he had scheduled or heads he needed to cut, they would wait. He made Jolene his priority as he walked out of the barbershop, jumped in his pickup truck, and drove thirty minutes to the pristine white hospital campus that felt like a city, within a city. Incubated unto itself in what would

have otherwise been a remote and wooded area, he met
Jolene in an open-air parking lot, since neither one of them
prepared ahead of time to pay the five dollars cash to park in
the garage.

They walked hand in hand with barely a word
between them on the tree-lined streets. Pine trees, oak trees,
and palm trees swung high in the air, ruffled by the light
breeze. Trees with indigo and red blossoms, jacarandas and
royal poincianas, added beauty and color to the green-scape,
and red mulch piled between shrubs added vibrancy to their
ruminative walk. Even if they wanted to dwell in the gray area
of ambiguity, their surroundings wouldn't allow it. The
greenery on their walk from the parking lot to the appointed
building wouldn't let them wallow in their misery. The live
plants and the back lit portraits of plants and fruits inside the
doctor's office, wouldn't let them remain miserly. Even the
carpet used throughout the building, instead of tile, provided
a warmth as they navigated hallways, and followed nurses to
their interior, windowless room, where they wait for what's to
come.

Her eyes are on him, his eyes focus on parts of her.
With heavy hooded lids he stares from her neck to her
breasts, up and down, wishing he could see through her green
blouse, waist trainer, body shaper, and bra, to her body.

This is ridiculous.

"This is ridiculous," Mosiah says.

"What, Babe." Jolene responds.

"They call you here, give you an appointment time,
and then make you wait forever."

"That's how it goes at every appointment. You're here
for an hour but only see the doctor for five minutes, and they
make all the money. Worse than lawyers and their damn
billable hours."

Mosiah goes back to brooding. His body rocks
slightly in the chair as he emits more sighs from the pit of his
gut.

She watches him thinking, *patience was never his specialty.
Always preferring to do something different, go somewhere else if he's not*

getting what he wants right when he wants it. He did that when I was with Jemarcus. He just had to be with Cindy, even though he left her at prom to come see me in the hospital to make sure I was all right.

"Sorry to keep you waiting," Doctor Richards says.

She breezes into the door and takes extra time to make sure it is securely shut behind her.

She says, "Thank you for coming in on such short notice."

"No problem," Jolene says. "This is my husband, Mosiah."

"Good afternoon. How are you?" Doctor Richards extends her hand.

Mosiah takes one hand down from his face to shake. "Good," he says. "Just waiting on you."

"Yes. Yes. Yes. So we have the results back from the biopsy and with the results of the MRI. . . there really is no easy way to say this . . . Mrs. Walker, you have breast cancer. Triple-negative. Stage four."

Jolene nods her head as she feels the walls close in around her until their painted coats touch her face. She nods in her boxed in space, doing the only thing she knows how. Her bumbling bobble head makes up for the lack of words she has to share. The lack of expression she has to offer. The lack of vocabulary she has to articulate the suffocating feeling filling her body. For Jolene, it is as if the air was vacuum sucked out of the room when Doctor Richards secured the door. She focuses on her stark white lab coat, ebullient against the pea green slacks, and navy blouse with the peter pan collar.

Breathe Jolene.

She puts her hands on the cushioned exam table beside where her hips sit and presses her weight into them. She folds over her legs. Her head dives first between her thighs propelling her body forward off of the table into Mosiah.

"Jo!"

He snaps her name as he catches her in his arms.

"Jo, Baby. Are you alright?"

"Sorry," she says.

Mosiah helps her stand and sit back on the table. He stands beside her, holding her hand. It is not the casual grasp they shared crossing the parking lot. Her hand grips his, her manicured nails dig into his skin. She uses him as her own pressure point, forcing all of her energy through her hand and nails into him to alleviate the breathlessness of her own consternation.

"What's next?" Mosiah asks.

"How long do I have?" Jolene asks.

"Jo, don't talk like that," Mosiah chastises.

"The cancer is aggressive," Doctor Richards says. "And it has spread. It's in your head, spine and legs."

"What's next?" Mosiah demands to know again.

"How long do I have?" Jolene insists.

"Mrs. Walker, there is no need to jump to conclusions," Doctor Richards says. "Mr. Walker, the next step is treatment. There's too much of it for surgery. So we can start with chemo and then radiation, and after that, we'll see where we are."

"When?" Mosiah asks.

"You'll have to schedule the appointment, but you should be able to get in for your first session soon."

"What about the study that says some breast cancer patients don't need chemo?" Jolene asks.

"That doesn't apply here. You're stage four."

"I saw it on the news. There were stage four patients not getting chemo and they got to keep their hair?"

"The study you're talking about is not being done here."

"Then where is it?"

"New York."

"JoJo, there are other treatments," Mosiah says.

"How . . . How did I . . . How did I get ca . . . ca . . . cancer?" Jolene ekes out.

Her voice is without its accented vibrancy and resilience. It is small and choked. Her body still searches for the rest of the air in the room. Her mind wonders how everyone is standing, talking, functioning, when her heart can't pump enough oxygenated blood to her brain to tell her legs not to wobble, her knees not to collapse, her body not to shake with a roll of shivers, or direct her mind to create a coherent sentence that doesn't sound like a child still learning to speak.

"Well," Doctor Richards begins. "African-American women and Hispanic women are more likely to develop triple-negative breast cancer. But beyond that, you were also a teen mom, and you're overweight. All of these are risk factors by themselves."

"So I was just the perfect storm of symptoms?"

Doctor Richards doesn't answer Jolene's rhetorical ringing bell. She pivots, "Like I said, you are definitely a candidate for chemo and radiation. That would be the biggest help right now. We can also see about getting you into a few clinical trials further down the road."

"No," Jolene says with the full force of her voice. "Absolutely not."

"Jo, just listen," Mosiah urges.

"No, Mo. I will not be their test dummy for medicine they don't even know works. I've already got a scar from a procedure I didn't need. We don't need to add, or do, anything else to me, or on me, in the name of science."

"Jolene. This is not the same as the C-section. Just listen."

"No. This ain't the forties. We're not in Tuskegee or Johns Hopkins. And my name ain't Henrietta Lacks. No."

"Jolene," Mosiah snaps.

"Mr. Walker, it's okay," Doctor Richards assuages. "Many patients, black women especially, feel like Mrs. Walker. But know that the treatment you were talking about for stage four patients who don't get chemo is a clinical trial. That's not a fully approved treatment. Just know that getting into a trial is something to think about down the road. It won't be today. It won't be tomorrow. Just later."

"Thank you," Mosiah says.

"I'm going to leave you two to talk," Doctor Richards says. "Take your time. There is no rush. When you're done, go to the front and give them your chart, and they'll get you right on the schedule for the chemo treatment in the Davis Building. The sooner the better."

Doctor Richards walks out of the exam room and shuts the door tightly behind her. Jolene, eyes blinded by the white coat of the departing doctor, releases Mosiah's hand. She brings both of her hands to her face. Warm tears drip over her fingertips as she tries to wipe them away as soon as they form. She has found her air. Enough of it to sigh as she cries. To cry until her cheeks and nose are wet, the latter secreting more mucus, covering her wiping fingers in the pitiable bodily fluid.

"How are we going to pay for this?" Jolene asks through her tears.

"You have insurance," Mosiah says.

"I have a basic plan to cover me you and the kids. I don't have a flex account with money just sitting in it waiting for somebody to be diagnosed with death."

"You're not going to die, Jolene."

"You don't know that," she says. "Stage four. Triple-negative. That's the stuff that makes headlines when basic white women end up dead. With my black ass face, nobody's going to care to make sure I'm treated with the best they have to offer."

"That's why we're here," Mosiah says. "That's why I made the appointment here. That's why I kept telling you to go to the doctor. You were too worried about everybody else when you should have been worrying about yourself. I told you."

"Okay, Mosiah. You told me. Now what?"

"I'll pick up a private plan. Obamacare is still around, right?"

"But now you know I have a pre-existing condition. That shit's going to be high as hell. I can't just go to the VA like you."

"Don't make it out like it's all that."

"And you want to get remarried. This is ironic."

"Jo, that's not important right now."

"In sickness and in health, 'til death do us part. It's coming sooner than we think."

"Jolene."

"What, Mo? What?"

"We can do both."

"How? We can't afford it. The only reason I'm going back to school, besides Granny Mae, is because it will help me get a raise at work. Teachers don't make no money, and you're still taking losses on your businesses."

"We're doing both, Jolene. We can do the vow renewal and the chemo and the radiation, and the trials, and whatever else we need to do."

"And we're going to be homeless by the end of it."

"Jolene. Stop worrying. Stop giving up. You haven't even started yet."

"Mosiah, she just issued me a death sentence. What do you mean, stop worrying? I haven't even started worrying yet."

"Jolene. We will face this."

"You're not facing anything, Mo. This is not Iraq, or Afghanistan, or wherever the hell you were. This is my life. I was born alone. I'm going to die alone."

"Jolene. Where do you want to get married?"

"What . . . What are you talking about?"

"Just answer the question. Where do you want to get married?"

"We're already married and we're not having the vow renewal service. We can't do both."

"Okay. Where did you want to get married when we first got married?"

"Huh? Why?"

"Just answer the question."

"Mo, you already know the answer."

"Answer the question, Jo."

"The beach."

"Then that's where we're doing the vow renewal. Let's go.

"Go where?"

"To the beach. We're picking a venue?"

"Mo. Stop. I know what you're trying to do. The only place I'm going is to make this appointment for chemo, and then I have to go and get Lydia and Toussaint from camp."

"I'll tell my dad to get the kids."

"You have to get back to the shop."

"I'll tell the guys to cover for me."

"Mosiah."

Jolene sighs. It is the only thing she can do. She has seen him when he's been like this before. Stubborn and obstinate, bull-headed and intractable, convinced that he can outrun, outsmart, and outgun whatever is in his way. It's what he wrote her in letter after letter, while he was away fighting, defending and protecting. He always signed the bottom of every letter, Mosiah Alan Walker, Master of my own Destiny. She recognized it as a proclamation to himself as much as it was a prophesy for the rest of his life.

Now he's determined to prophesy over her; fighting, winning, defeating the enemy called cancer, and celebrating with a victory marriage.

"Give me your hand," Mosiah says.

"For what?"

"Damnit, Jo. Just give me your hand."

"Ugh. Fine."

She places her hand in his. He pulls her down off the table to the floor.

"Look at me," he says lifting her chin.

She sees calm where worry was written just minutes earlier.

Mosiah says, "I promised to provide and protect, to support and defend you against all enemies."

"Mosiah, that's the marine oath."

"They were also my vows to you."

"We don't have time for this. Let's go," she says, pulling his hand.

He holds her back. He holds her until she turns around and looks at him, all of him. The black polo shirt, dark denim jeans, freshly edged hair, the trimmed goatee of his growing beard, and the fiery determination in his eyes. He holds her hand until she shifts the weight in her feet, anxious to leave, anxious to move onto what's next, anxious to be left alone resigned to her fate, without a possibility of a forward future.

"You will get well and we're getting remarried."

"Okay, Mosiah."

"You have to believe that."

"Okay, I believe it. Can we go now?"

"Let's go. Make your appointment, and then we're going to the beach."

"Whatever, Mosiah."

"It's not whatever. It's forever."

Jolene smiles, "You are so damn corny."

"But you love me anyway."

"Let's go, Mo."

"Mojo getting married. Mojo getting married. Mojo getting married."

Mosiah chants behind Jolene as they walk to the front of the office. He chants to keep her smiling, to keep her on the precipice of laughter. He adds a shoulder shimmy and a high step as they wait at the counter to keep her mind on him, and off of the appointment she's making. He chants and dances from the white office building to the paved lot, where they both parked. He is her jester until she is in the SUV with the door closed. He walks around his truck and gets inside. The engine hums at the turn of the ignition. Air blows and becomes cool. He turns the vents directly to his face and backs out of his space. Glancing in his rearview mirror, he drives forward, leading Jolene away from the city designed to deal with those suffering from infirmity. He only glances, not wanting her to see his eyes, as they sweat with the feelings he had to hide to convince her of the healing he's not sure any doctor can provide.

16.

Waiting at the light to exit the hospital campus Mosiah calls Jolene. He asks, "You wanna go to One Ocean?"

"You're just trying to spend all your money," Jolene says.

"Nah. But let's just go see."

"I'm following you."

Mosiah hangs up the phone and makes a left on Beach Boulevard onto A1A. He looks up in his rearview mirror to make sure Jolene is following behind him. They drive the quaint state road hugging the coast until they get to Atlantic Boulevard, where the luxury spa and resort rises in front of them. Mosiah narrows his eyes as he turns on Atlantic, hunting for a parking space, a meter, or a spot in the lot of the busy Beaches Town Center. It is the answer by Jacksonville's three beach communities to the massive town center complex across the Intracoastal waterway. Instead of taking the bridge across the ditch, everyone living on the expensive side of the water crowds into the small outdoor mall where the clothing options are linen, bathing suits, or board shorts, and the food options all proffer to visitors dining on the fresh catch of the day from the ocean, just miles away.

Mosiah lucks up and finds two spaces in the pay lot of the shopping complex. He blocks both spaces with his pick-up truck until Jolene drives from behind him to take one that four other drivers also saw in the hunt for a spot. He backs up just enough, giving Jolene room to pull in her SUV. Backing into the adjacent space next to her, he sees the four angry drivers pass him, glaring with anger that he took what should've been theirs.

Out in the open air, the wet, salty smell from the ocean barrages their senses. It is the reason most people who live at the beach say they moved across the ditch in the first place. The fresh smell of the ocean and the sound of the crashing waves, makes you feel like you're in an entirely different world, where time is limitless and work never calls. This part of the beach creates permanent vacation vibes for everyone who lives and works in the area. A marked difference from the atmosphere just twelve miles west in downtown Jacksonville where the homeless populate the city parks, the tall buildings are mostly vacant, and the only attraction worth traveling for is a Jaguars football game and maybe a concert at the arena, the amphitheater, or one of the concert halls.

"You ready?" Mosiah asks, waiting in front of her door.

"Yeah," Jolene says. "Let's go."

Mosiah walks to Jolene and grabs her hand. She slams the door shut and they walk together toward the rebuilt dunes where the sand oats and other vegetation are still taking root after being obliterated by back to back hurricanes two years in a row. Mosiah and Jolene walk from the outskirts of the property for the beachfront resort around to the front of the hotel, where its name is lit on a silver backdrop shaped like a wave with a fountain rising out of its top. They pass cars pulling up to the front for valet service and enter the sliding glass doors. They are immediately enveloped by the cool air offering a welcome relief to them and a group of over-tanned, overzealous bougie beach bums.

They are confronted by an atmosphere of opulence including marble floors, a grand marble staircase, and chandeliers of all shapes, kinds, and sizes.

Jolene says, "Having a vow renewal here easily costs fifty-thousand dollars."

"Probably," Mosiah says. "But it doesn't hurt to dream. They've made sure they have the best spot on the beach. Plus, we can do everything right here and never even leave."

"Mo, we can't afford this. You can look around the lobby and see we can even afford to stay here half a night in a regular room, let alone invite folks to come and spend the night and stay for a few days."

"Jolene, we're just looking," Mosiah says.

"There's a whole beach we can look at, you know."

"Where do you want to go?"

"Casa Marina."

"Can we at least take a tour here first?"

"For what?"

"So we don't look lost walking in and walking right back out. You see all these people staring at us because we haven't moved from the entrance, we look like we don't belong."

"I don't care what these people think."

"May I help you?" A woman says, walking up to Mosiah and Jolene.

"No, thank you," Jolene says. "We were just leaving."

"Actually, I have a question," Mosiah says.

"I'd be happy to help you, sir. I'm Maritza, the concierge specialist here at One Ocean."

Jolene rolls her eyes at the woman walking around in red bottom pumps to work as a glorified greeter at the hotel. She lags behind Mosiah, holding his hand, gently tugging him toward the sliding glass doors every other second. He ignores her urging and lingers in front of the mixed race woman. He takes in the color of her tanned skin with hair flowing in voluminous curls down to her waist, surmising that she grew up speaking Spanish and Creole.

"I'm Mosiah," he says. "My wife and I want to renew our vows and we wanted to know if that is something we can do here."

"Yes. Absolutely. One Ocean is the premiere destination for weddings, honeymoons, and even a staycation when you just want to get away."

"So we've been told," Jolene says.

"Yes," Maritza says. "If you have a moment, you can look through our gallery at some of the weddings we've done here. And we can take you on a tour of the grounds and look at the menu to see what you might like."

"That sounds good," Mosiah says with an eager smile. "Doesn't it, Jo? Doesn't that sound good?"

Jolene asks, "How much does the average wedding here run?"

"It depends on your number of guests and what services you'd like to have. We can go as big or as small as you'd like."

"Let's say fifty guests with all the bells and whistles. Plated dinner with the option of steak, chicken, or fish. Open top-shelf bar, flowers, candles, band, the works."

"Well, ma'am," Maritza says. "I don't know right off the top of my head, but that could be upwards of seventy-five thousand dollars . . . and that's a conservative estimate."

"Exactly. Thank you for your time," Jolene says. "Come on, Mo."

"Thank you," Mosiah says, as he allows Jolene to drag him out of the door.

Outside, they walk quickly away from the hotel back to the lot where they wasted four dollars to park. Jolene seethes as she paces the pressure washed streets.

I don't know what's gotten into him, but he acts like we didn't just leave the doctor's office.

Mosiah let's her stew in her own irrational anger. He hums as he goes, a light, made up tune that keeps a bop in his step until they get to their cars. Jolene chirps her alarm and rushes to the driver's side door to open it for herself. Mosiah shrugs and walks to his pickup truck. By the time he's started his ignition, Jolene is backing out with her window down.

She yells at him, "Follow me."

Jolene navigates her way out of the parking lot and back on to the street. She doesn't check her rearview mirror to make sure Mosiah is behind her. She can hear the steady rumble of his truck as they drive block for block on A1A, away from the upscale and sadiddy surroundings of One Ocean and Atlantic Beach to the more affordable and accessible area of Jacksonville Beach. The small seaside community is in the middle of four others, each one with an increased cost compared to the last. To the north there is Neptune Beach and then Atlantic Beach, and to the south there is St. Augustine Beach and Ponte Vedra Beach. In the middle, at Jax Beach, is the community for families who just found out they were well-to-do and could afford ocean adjacent property.

Jolene drives until the boutiques and scratch kitchen restaurants give way to strip malls with recognizable store names and franchised chain restaurants. It is here, in the middle of everything that can be found on the other side of the ditch, that Jolene pulls into the wrought iron fenced in parking lot of the rustic white building erected in 1925. They find five dollar side-by-side parking spaces immediately. Outside Mosiah sees Jolene's mood has automatically picked up from the surly and resistant attitude she had two beach cities away.

He says, "Just because it's old doesn't mean it's going to be cheaper."

"Maybe not, but you got me out here, and this is the place I want to see."

"After you," Mosiah says.

He watches Jolene bound toward the stucco building in the spanish-mediterannean style of the era it was built in. It is the first time he's seen her this buoyant in weeks. *It worked* he thinks to himself. He pretends to be as averse to going inside the boutique hotel and restaurant as she was to going inside the bombastic grandeur of One Ocean. He pouts behind her until she turns around and sees his face.

Jolene says, "C'mon. We're just looking,"

"There's a whole beach we can look at, you know."

"Come. On."

"Alright, alright."

Mosiah picks up his pace to keep up with Jolene. He tries to hide the smile exploding on the inside of him.

If I can keep her smiling and focused on this, on us, she won't have to think about her diagnosis.

"Good afternoon, are you dining in?" the hostess asks from behind a black podium.

"No," Jolene says. "We'd like to get a quote about doing our vow renewal here."

"Let me get the person who does weddings here. It'll be just a moment."

The woman disappears from the hostess stand. Jolene and Mosiah wait just inside the doors of the restaurant that is larger on the inside than it appears from outside.

She says, "Isn't this cute?"

"It's alright. It's old."

"But that's what makes it charming."

"Look who's finally ready to get remarried."

Jolene looks up at him and rolls her eyes. She says, "You told me to dream. So I'm dreaming. I've always wanted to get married here. Even the first time when we didn't have no money."

"Why didn't you ever say anything?" Mosiah asks.

"What would have been the point. I was just out of school and so were you. I had Toussaint and you were still trying to build up your base at the shop. Besides, you know your dad would have rung both of our necks if we didn't have a church wedding."

"He could have still presided over the ceremony if you wanted to be on the beach."

"Mo, it's not a big deal. The first time was for our family. This time it's for us."

Thank you, God, Mosiah says in a quick internal prayer. *It's been a long time since she's been this optimistic. Has she ever been this optimistic?*

He dismisses the unintended question thrust on him by his subconscious. He says, "Let's make it all about us."

Mosiah looks down on her and smiles. Jolene presses her lips together and smiles right back. She gives him what he needs to see; her at ease. She curates the facade she knows he's been trying to pull out of her the best way he knows how; optimism, distraction and positive reinforcement. She play acts the role, not letting him see the unease coursing through her body after being diagnosed with a terminal disease.

The doctor didn't give me a time but that doesn't mean the clock hasn't started. According to her, it's been started.

"Hello, I'm Ross Buchanan, the wedding concierge here at Casa Marina. How may I help you?"

"I'm Jolene and this is my husband, Mosiah, and we're looking to get our vows renewed."

"How you doin'," Mosiah says, waving a hand at the tall, lanky white man in a sea foam green button down, and seersucker slacks.

"That's awesome," Ross says. "When is your anniversary?"

"March ninth," Jolene answers.

"And how long have you guys been married?"

"Six years. Going on seven," Mosiah says.

"Lucky number seven," Ross says. "Well, come this way and we can talk about the number of guests and if anyone will be staying or not."

"We're thinking like fifty guests, but probably only overnight accommodations for us," Mosiah says.

"That's great. That's great," Ross says. "Well, right out here is where we have most of our ceremonies. It's great because you're out in the beach atmosphere, but not right down on the sand, so you don't have to worry about getting dirty and getting the sand everywhere."

"This is beautiful," Jolene says.

She walks through the attached veranda at the back of the building. She crosses the elevated stage where she's seen brides, grooms and their officiants stand in ceremony after ceremony in the venue's online gallery, and walks to the gates enclosing the property. She looks out over the dunes to the ocean.

"These gates can open for pictures on the walkover," Ross says, walking up behind Jolene. "Or if you want to go right down to the beach you can."

"Thank you," she says.

"Your anniversary is on a Saturday, so if you guys want to lock this date in now we can, and I'll put together a couple estimates for you. We can do either a traditional dinner wedding, an afternoon, or a sunrise breakfast/brunch type of wedding."

"That's different," Jolene says, still staring out over the water.

"That'll be great," Mosiah says, coming to stand beside Jolene. "Thanks, man."

"I'll be right back with those numbers."

Ross walks away leaving Jolene and Mosiah alone on the clean, pergola covered courtyard, a gateway away from the power of the Atlantic.

"What do you think?" Jolene asks.

"Is this what you want."

If I live long enough. "Yes," she answers.

This is what I've always wanted. When I thought Jemarcus and I were going to get married; we used to plan our future in the back of his sex-funky Pontiac. We were going to get engaged after graduation, like the high school couples from nineties teen sitcoms, and get married. I used to search for wedding venues in my journalism class when I was supposed to be writing articles for the newspaper. Then I was pregnant, and then he dumped me, and then there was Franchesca, and then there was you. Mosiah. There was always you.

Jolene turns to look at him. His brow is relaxed and his face is tranquil and content. She tries to mirror his image, to match his serenity.

"This is it," he says, taking her hand in his.

Jolene turns to look at Mosiah. She knows he is trying to keep her happy, distracted, and upbeat, instead of wallowing in self-pitying deprecation. She looks at the profile of his face as gratitude replaces the cancer-induced worry pumping through her veins.

She says, "Thank you."

They look out over the beachfront property at the young white families, chasing toddlers under pop-up tents, and rainbow umbrellas. Jolene watches one couple chase a little girl about Lydia's age, back and forth across the sand. They run through a warming tide pool left by the receding high tide. Jolene can see the water splash as she imagines the shrieks and laughters coming from the mother, father, and little girl. Mosiah locks in on where Jolene gazes. He sees what she sees. The family, the joy, the moment in time when their life is truly carefree. He looks down at Jolene. Her thick hair is perfectly framed around her face, the spaghetti strap, yellow sundress blows away from her body. He looks at her from the crown of her head to her toes, painted purple, and knows she is looking out over the ocean in prayer. Her eyes are open but her gaze is set beyond the family that conjured up images of her own children, into something further he can not see. He looks out into the deep blue depths of the boundless, endless saltwater and prays on his own.

Dear God. Make this work.

His prayer is simple and to the point. Where his father could take a text and preach a whole sermon, start a prayer and have people shouting in a moment, Mosiah never could. Despite his name, and his father's urging, he never felt or heard the call, the conviction to lead and take over the church. It is the reason he went to the military, to avoid bible college, lessons in Greek and Hebrew and the seminary. He fought to escape, and when he came home he chose to cut hair and clean because he'd seen too much of what the world really looks like to try to step into the pulpit and preach provision and prosperity. He stuck with his mother's gift, ministering to himself with music; a song always in his mind, a tune forever in the hum of his lips.

He hums the famous gospel song by Tata Vega as Jolene stares in prayer. The hymn that created a joyful end to a melancholy movie, based on a book about the beauty of the color purple. Mosiah hums until Jolene snaps out of her trance and turns to him.

She says, "What are we going to tell Toussaint and Lydia?"

"She's too young to understand," Mosiah says.

"Toussaint isn't."

"Let's wait," Mosiah says.

"He's going to know," Jolene says. "He's going to know something is wrong with me."

"Toussaint is just a kid. He's so wrapped up in his own world, he won't even be paying attention."

Jolene nods. "If he asks me, I'm going to tell him."

"Okay, Baby. Okay."

Mosiah knows better than to fight with Jolene about Toussaint. A lesson he learned early on in their relationship. Even though he adopted him, gave him his last name, TeeTee was still her son. Her first born. Her Toussaint. The boy she named from a poem she loved in a book about the suffering, survival, and success of color coated women like her.

"Alright guys," Ross says, coming out of the doors of the restaurant, back onto the patio. "I've got a few different options worked up for you here."

"We'll take it," Mosiah says, taking the paper from Ross' hand.

"That's great. That's great," Ross says. He shows off the over eager smile he's been trying to suppress since they arrived. "What time slot would you like?"

"Sunrise," Jolene says. "I want to say "I do" the moment the moon goes down and the sun comes up with the light of a new day."

"That's great. Now the ninth is the day before the spring forward for daylight savings time, so you may have to wake up early to catch the sun."

"Thank you," Jolene says.

"Well, I have all the information you need right here. If you want we can do the deposit now, and lock everything in, or if you need to take a moment and call us back, I'll hold you on the schedule for a week before I have to release the date."

"We'll lock it in now," Mosiah says. "We know what we want."

"Alright," Ross says. "Let's do it. Just follow me inside to my office and we'll get you folks squared away. Let's have us a wedding."

Ross laughs with the nervous excitement of someone who knows they've overstepped their bounds, but is too exuberant to care or contain themselves. Mosiah and Jolene follow him away from the ocean, away from the beach, away from the frolicking families in the surf, away from the place where they will stand in nine months to say, "I do" again.

They follow Ross and his excitement away from the prayers they prayed to the God they were both raised to know.

His, *Dear God. Make this work.*

Hers, *Dear God. Let me live to live my dream.*

17.

Stacks of magazines are piled around Jolene in her room on the eighth floor of the Davis Building at the Mayo clinic campus. She sits in one of the leather recliners in a room of the chemo ward. Natural sunlight streams in from the window with the open blinds behind her. Machines and stands with machines surround her, ready to monitor her vital signs and the progress of her first three hour treatment. She is alone in the room, waiting for the nurse to come in and administer, the treatment that has a distinct sanitizing smell with lingering notes of mint. She is alone as she requested to be. She told Tanya and Vaughn to go to work. She told Mosiah to keep his clients at the shop, and the contracts for his cleaning company. She told her parents to remain in retirement. She told them she wanted the first experience to be her own, and she would report back on whether they could accompany her on any of the other five treatments in the plan.

Her journal is in her lap. The soft leather bound book of her thoughts is open and the pen is in her hand. She wants to write but she hesitates. Jolene is reluctant to put her thoughts down on paper, knowing they could very well be some of her last. Her own mortality facing her, she is reticent to document the experience of what she faces that could live on in perpetuity, for all posterity. Lydia and Toussaint's faces come clear into her mind. She can see them with the journal that's in her lap sitting between them. She sees Toussaint reading it to Lydia, while Mosiah observes from a discreet distance away. He too listening, rapt with intent trying to uncover the makings of the wife he lost to a disease he couldn't will or pray away.

Jolene's thoughts descend into a vision of what her life looks like without her in it. Sitting straight up in the well-used chemo recliner, her journal in her lap, books and magazines at her feet, Jolene sees her daughter forgetting her, her son reminding her of the mommy he knew first, and her husband eventually moving on to the next woman. A woman he picks on purpose because she looks nothing like the dead wife he will always love. Jolene imagines the new woman, the new wife that will take over for her when she is gone. A chocolate woman with clear skin the color of night, a thin body, and a sing-song voice that assuages any concerns that she can't hold a candle to the woman she is replacing. Jolene imagines a white woman by Mosiah's side; a blonde hair, blue eyed WASP. The waspiest of all the WASPs that have ever WASPed. A woman who likes to run and bike for fun, even in the cold, and who will look on with a tight smile in Mosiah's father's church as he preaches blessings and salvation, and brimstone and hell fire in the same message, and sometimes in the same breath. She imagines Mosiah enjoying the freedom that comes with being with a woman who can get her hair wet whenever and doesn't wear a scarf. The new wife will be fascinated by the unruly kinks and curls of Lydia's mane, that don't comply when water is applied.

Jolene imagines the wedding between Mosiah and the new woman. The wedding she planned for them at Casa Marina. The beachside ceremony and brunch she dreamed about having with Jemarcus when she was sixteen, before she knew the meaning of marriage.

July 11,

It's funny how things work out in life. Or how God works them out, because this isn't anything I would choose for me. I daydream about all the things I want, all the grand plans, and ideas I have, all the vacations I want to take, and I can't even experience them. I'm dreaming dreams for somebody else. I guess this is how Moses felt looking out over the promised land, knowing he would never get there with the Israelites he led forever. How Dr. King knew one day there would be a black president, even though he'd never live to see it. I'm not saying I'm Moses or King, but I mean every woman should get to live out the wedding of her dreams. At least once, right?

"Good morning, Mrs. Walker," a nurse says walking into the room. "Sorry to keep you waiting; we were getting everything setup for you."

"Don't worry about it. I've got nowhere else to be and plenty to keep me entertained."

"I see," the nurse says, looking at Jolene's stacks of books. "Who's getting married?"

"It's supposed to be me," Jolene says. "My husband and I want to renew our vows next year."

"That's great . . ."

"But we have to get through this first."

"You will, because now you have something to look forward to," the nurse says. "Let's get you set up."

The short nurse in baby blue scrubs, sporting a deep chocolate colored bob wig, begins to hookup the devices. She rolls them closer to Jolene's recliner and sets up the IV of the curing poisonous drip.

"Roll up your sleeve for me, please," the nurse says. "Oh, that's a pretty color for your sweater. That yellow looks good on you."

"Thank you. When I'm feeling a kind of way, I try to be intentional in dressing the opposite."

The nurse, bent at the waist, focuses on taping Jolene's arm to insert the IV. She says, "A little reverse psychology there. I'm sure it helps."

"Sometimes."

The nurse stands up between Jolene and the monitors. "Okay, Mrs. Walker, we're going to start pushing the chemo through the IV."

"Okay."

"Do you have any questions before we get started?"

"No."

"Just so you're aware, you're going to feel a sensation coursing through your body when it first starts going in. It will dissipate after a while. If it's too much for you we can slow it down."

"Let's get this over with," Jolene says.

"Alright, try to make yourself comfortable."

"I've got enough reading to keep me company."

"It's going in now, Mrs. Walker."

Jolene nods as she reaches over to pick up one of the wedding books Mosiah dropped off with her. She has a book on floral arrangements, cakes, cuisine, and at least three on wedding gowns. She picks up the one dedicated to flowers and other creative decorations. The book representing the opposite of everything she currently has.

"Get rid of all your plants," Doctor Richards told her in a follow-up phone call. "And start eating canned vegetables and canned fruit."

"Why," Jolene asked.

"We can't risk you getting sick from a parasite or anything that comes on fresh food. Yes it's better for you, but when you're being treated with chemo it actually makes things worse," Doctor Richards said.

Jolene opens the magazine as she feels warmth sweeping her lower body. It's concentrated in her lap. There is warmth, there is sensation, there is tingling.

She gasps with her mouth opened into an elongated O. "That's different," Jolene says out loud.

"It'll pass, Mrs. Walker," the nurse says, monitoring the machinery pumping the drug.

"I'd never thought it'd feel like this. Y'all should have taken me on a date first before this."

The nurse bursts out laughing.

Jolene continues, "Y'all got me in here feeling like I don't know whether I should stay still for treatment, or go home, find my man, and get us both off."

The nurse continues laughing. Through her bursts of joy she says, "Mrs. Walker, I can slow down how much you're getting at once, if you feel uncomfortable."

"I don't know if uncomfortable is the right word. More like exposed."

"Just ride it out."

"That's what I tell my husband."

The nurse laughs again. The vocal rejoicing Jolene knows comes from deep within her belly makes her crack a smile of her own. It is genuine and unforced. It begins as a smirk creeping up one side of her mouth before spreading across her face.

"Mrs. Walker, you've got me crying real tears back here."

"Crying is not what I was feeling like doing. But I guess what I felt would be inappropriate since we're in such a public place."

"It'll pass," the nurse says through a chuckle.

"It's passing alright."

"Some people describe it as feeling like they have something crawling over them, or ants in their pants."

"That's one way to put it, but it's better now."

"Good," the nurse says, coming around to face Jolene. "Do you need anything?"

"Nope. I've got everything I need. I'll probably take a nap."

"We'll be in and out to check on you, and we have water and snacks as well."

"Thank you."

"See you in a bit, Mrs. Walker."

Jolene watches the nurse leave her room. She leaves her to her journal and the book of flowers in her lap. Jolene opens the book and flips through page after page of floral arrangements. She takes mental notes of the ones she likes, her preference for the bouquets of lilies over the ones that have mostly roses. She knows she wants colors, instead of mostly white, and lots of greenery. Ivy and magnolia leaves used as accent pieces with pops of color from a few sparsely populated flowers are the ones she marks. The waxy leaves are strung together to create garland, wreaths, or used as crowns for brides and flower girls alike.

That's pretty.

Jolene comes to a page in the book with a black bride and groom posed in a circle of gardenia flowers. She stares at the model couple, wondering if they're really married. If the image captured and stamped into the book is really a snapshot of their love or the beautiful eye of the photographer capturing an idea to spur someone else's reality. Jolene looks at the couple in the image and gives them names. She assigns them personalities and traits to carry them through their love that will be a story for the ages. She imagines the bride old and wrinkly, laying in a hospital bed beside her groom who is old and deaf in one ear. She imagines them holding hands through the rails of their bed, crying when the other has to leave to be bathed, or examined or treated.

Jolene pulls her phone from where she tucked it into the side pocket of the recliner. It alights to life in her hand. She opens the camera, snaps a picture of the picture, and sends it to Mosiah.

If I make it I want to do this

Jolene goes back to the book. She turns the page on the couple girded by gardenias, exuding happily ever after to another grouping of floral arrangements. Her phone vibrates and dings with a message.

Don't say if. You will make it.
I'll be there in a couple hours to pick you up.

Jolene sighs. She closes the book of flowers and puts her journal on top of it. She opens the page to where she left off and re-reads her lament before putting her pen back to the paper.

I wish I could be what he is to me. Ever the positive reinforcement. I wish I had that kind of faith in him. In us. In God. Hell, in myself. Maybe that's why I'm restless. Wanna leave him before he leaves me. Before he realizes I'm just surviving on promises I made Granny Mae, and I'm a distraction that fell in his way.

I'm thirty years old with stage four breast cancer. If that's not his God moving me out of the way so he can live his life, I don't know what it is. I've been his distraction since we were kids. I don't have much longer left. The doctor said the average life span with treatment is thirteen months. I'll go easy and he won't even miss me. He can have the Casa Marina wedding with his new wife.

Stop thinking negative

The message comes in from Mosiah. It is a command. Jolene hovers her fingers over the keys to lie and say she wasn't thinking negatively. She wants to put up a front, but she knows it is futile. Jolene darkens the phone, flips the switch to put it on vibrate only, and drops it back in the side pocket of the worn, brown leather chemo recliner. She pulls the lever to elevate her feet and recline the back. Closing her journal, she leaves it in her lap and sets the book of flowers on top of the stack of other reading materials she won't open. Jolene closes her eyes and inhales the minty poison coursing through her veins to make her well.

Stop thinking negative.

Jolene conjures his voice to add weight to the demand, but she can't recall the tone or timbre. All that comes forth is the image of the brown bride from the circle of gardenia's standing next to Mosiah on beachfront property waiting to say "I do."

18.

"Knock, knock," Mosiah says, entering Jolene's room.

She is asleep in the recliner when he walks in. Her yellow sweater is pulled tightly across her neck and chest. The magazines he sent her with are scattered around her feet. The leather journal and pen he knows she totes with her everywhere is closed in her lap, her hand holds the page where she left off. He approaches her and grabs the journal to move it away.

"What are you doing?" Jolene asks groggily.

"I thought you were sleeping," Mosiah says. "I was just moving this out of the way for you."

"I got it," Jolene says, gripping her journal tightly. *What's that about?*

Mosiah shakes his head and dismisses her defensiveness as she tugs the journal away from his hands, and tucks it beside her jean clad thigh.

"The nurse says you're all done," Mosiah says. "How do you feel?"

"I feel okay right now," Jolene says. "Better than I'd thought I'd feel seeing as how I just pumped poison in my body to make me better."

"Can you stand?" Mosiah asks.

"She has to come and take the IV out."

"She already did."

Jolene pulls up the sleeve on her right arm and sees she is no longer attached to the machines monitoring her intake of the drug they hope kills the cancer in her body, without it killing her first.

"Give me your hand," Mosiah says.

"I got it, Mo."

He doesn't insist. He hovers closely to make sure she is steady on her feet, but he doesn't intrude or persist in having his own way. Jolene stands with relative ease and begins adjusting her clothes. He takes sidelong glances at her as he watches her play with the lay of her T-shirt, the rise of her jeans, and the hang of her sweater around the curves of her body. He can tell she is not wearing three layers of underclothes; that today she gave up on the Spanx and the waist trainer, and just let her muffin top roll the way it wanted to. He looks at her, longing to reach out and grab the thickness he can hold in his hands; all of her that keeps him connected when he is near. He decides against his instinct and picks up the books and magazines from the floor instead. He holds them, watching while she runs her fingers through her hair. She rakes through the thick straightened strands, with her fingers. He knows it is more her love letter of goodbye to the hair she's going to lose than it is any method to appropriately frame her face.

My crown and my glory, Mo. I'm going to lose it all.

That's what she said to him last night before going to bed. Staring in the mirror of the vanity set pressed against a wall in the bedroom, she oiled her scalp and began to cry over the hair that was still rooted to her head. Tears fell as she parted and applied Jamaican Black Castor Oil from an applicator bottle. In their room, he sat behind her on the bed and watched. He left her the space for her own solace, but remained close enough to comfort her in case she needed him. He watched her as she raked the comb through her hair and wrapped the luscious strands around her head. She raked and smoothed her hand, sealing in the moisture and the path of her comb until she was done. The gravity of her nightly routine that would soon become moot and obsolete hit him as he watched her take her time to meticulously tie the satin scarf that would hold her hair in place. He heard her ask herself, "How long will it take to fall out? How long do I have before I'm bald?"

To him she asked, "Do you think I will look good bald."

"You will look good no matter what," he said, holding himself.

"I've never been bald in my life. Not even as a baby."

Jolene, stared at herself in the mirror, examining her face, trying to imagine what she would be like, who she would be, without all the long pretty hair she was known for. The hair she thought made up for her extra inches and added pounds because it was all hers.

Mosiah looks at her in the hospital recliner the way he looked at her the night before. Only now she stares into space holding the freshly clipped ends of her hair, caressing the strands that will eventually shed and fall in the name of regenerative healing. Despite the books in his hands, his arms are wrapped around his body, holding himself tightly.

"You ready?" Mosiah asks in a cracking voice.

"Yeah, I'm ready."

Jolene walks to the recliner and grabs her purse and journal, and shoves it inside. Mosiah holds out his free hand to her. She takes it. They walk out of the room united against the common enemy they call cancer. He walks with her through the carpeted halls where door after door is either opened or closed, the electric light coding system mounted above each door, blinking the color for which stage of care each patient is in.

"Where do you want to go?" Mosiah asks.

"Home. I want to hang out with Lydia and Toussaint today while I have the energy. Doctor Richards says the first day you'll typically feel fine, but it's the second day you'll start to feel the affects of the medicine."

"We may need to make a stop first," Mosiah says.

"Where? Why?"

"Your parents want to see you. Your sisters too."

"They have cars. They can come to me."

"Granny Mae too."

"She's the only reason. You should've said her name first."

"I know, but everybody else wants to see you too."

"Let's go." Jolene sighs.

"Lydia and Toussaint are already there," Mosiah adds.

"So we were going to have to stop by and say "hey" no matter what I wanted? Why even make it seem like I had a choice in the matter?"

"Because now I know that once we get there, we don't have to stay all day and night. You know how your family gets."

Jolene smiles, "True."

They stop by the appointment desk and schedule Jolene for her next round of chemo before heading out to the lobby. On the elevator to the ground floor Jolene grips Mosiah's hand and lays her head on his shoulder. They are alone in the enclosed space. Their thoughts their own, unshared with the partner beside them. The elevator hums around them as seven floors go by in a matter of seconds. They don't stop for anyone to get on and descend with them. Mosiah and Jolene arrive on the first floor hand in hand, the double doors of the elevators opening on the future in front of them. Jolene straightens up and walks with Mosiah down the long carpeted hallways with potted greenery and framed art all around them, to the parking garage where he left her SUV. He feels the tension in her body as he helps her up into her seat. Jolene waits until the medical campus is behind them, until she can no longer see the official signage, to relax.

One appointment down. Five more to go.

She stares out of the windshield as San Pablo Road feeds into JTB. She let's the road of the highway mesmerize her mind into nothingness. She lays her head against the interior of the door and closes her eyes. Mosiah steals glances at her until she appears to be sleep. It is then he feels the tension leave his own body. The tension he absorbed from her, tension he held because he pretended to be calm when he wasn't; feigning an illustration of relaxation that he wasn't. In the room, through the halls, in the elevators, out the door, through the parking garage, he longed to ask her questions he wasn't sure she was ready to answer. He longed to know about the entire three-hour experience she would have to repeat five more times. He wanted to know how she felt on the inside. Did she feel better already? But he knew she was in no place to play twenty questions.

He steals glances every few miles waiting, wanting to see her wake up and be different. He wants to know if he's still got the same girl, or if the prognosis of her health has transformed her into a woman he will no longer recognize. A woman whose soul will no longer be perfectly aligned to his. Mosiah drives from highway to highway until he's back to their beginning. The neighborhood that raised them, the blocks that made them, the schools where they met, and the homes that nurtured them. When Mosiah pulls up in front of the Lewis family home it is not long before the front door is burst open wide, and Lydia is bounding down the steps. Toussaint follows her. Mosiah looks at him, the son who belongs to him in name only. The son he told the truth despite his promise to Jolene.

"She's fine," Mosiah mouths to him.

He can see him relax as well. Mosiah can see the invisible weight partially lift from his fourteen year old shoulders. He walks around to the passenger side and opens Jolene's door.

"C'mon, Baby, we're here," Mosiah says.

"Where," Jolene asks.

"Your mom and dad's."

"Where are they?"

"Inside. Everybody is inside."

"Not me, Daddy," Lydia says. "I right here."

"Girl, get out the street," Jolene scolds quickly.

"Mommy, pick me up." Lydia demands.

"Mommy can't pick you up," Mosiah says. "She's tired."

"Daddy, pick me up," Lydia says.

"I can't. Daddy has to help Mommy"

"Toussaint," Jolene yells. "Come get your sister out the street."

Hearing his mother's voice come out clear, loud, and strong, Toussaint runs from where he stopped on the steps of the embankment down to the curb. He runs to where Jolene, Mosiah, and Lydia are huddled. What he sees encourages him even more. His mother, standing upright looking like her normal self, Mosiah holding her hand, Lydia being annoying begging them to pick her up.

She doesn't look sick, he thinks to himself.

"Get your sister, boy, and stop standing there like a deer in headlights," Jolene yells.

"Ugh, come here," Toussaint yells at Lydia.

"TeeTee, pick me up." She thrusts her arms in the air in front of him.

He hoists her into his arms and walks around the car to the curb. Mosiah watches him the whole way, seeing his shoulders relaxed on his back, his face a scowl of disdain for having to hold his sister. The look of concern that was on his face when he ran out of the front door a phantom that has long past.

Mosiah walks with Jolene around the front of the SUV, up the stairs, and into the unlocked doors of her parents' house. When they walk inside, her entire family greets them from either the dining room or the adjacent living room.

Their words rush at her at once. All a variation of, "Hey, Jo, how you feel? How you doing? You alright? You want something to eat?"

She takes the lead, even though she's holding on to Mosiah's hand, and guides them out of the way of the spotlight made just for her. She walks past her family in the living and dining rooms and heads for the small kitchen behind the wall. She sits down at the small round table in the seat that has always been hers, lays her head against the fading oil-stained wallpaper, and rests.

"You sure you want to sit in here?" Mosiah asks. "You know everybody is waiting on you. Waiting to see how you're doing."

"I barely know how I'm doing. All I want to do is go home. You said we had to come here to get the kids. So I'm here."

"Well, what do you want me to tell them?" Mosiah asks.

"Tell them whatever you want to tell them. Tell them the truth. I'm tired. I want to go home."

"Alright, Jo. Alright."

Mosiah walks out of the kitchen, leaving Jolene alone as she requested in the house that used to be her home. She briefly opens her eyes to take in the space. It is spotlessly clean, even the bell wallpaper behind the sink and counter shines. She closes her eyes, rests her head against the wall and sighs. Her heaviness doesn't lift as her ears pick up the increasingly loud murmur of the voices in the living room. The whispered questions of, "Is she alright?" passing back and forth from the eldest voice to the youngest voice. She hears Mosiah's clipped, "she's fine," in response. "She's just tired," he explains. Mumbles continue around the room, but she can imagine them nodding their heads and shifting uncomfortably in the awkward silence that begins to fall as they each question internally whether they should come and check on her or let her be. Jolene waits in the kitchen for whoever will arrive first. The one they will designate to break the ice. She waits for Vaughn. It's always Vaughn. The sister who inserts herself into everything, involving everyone, all the time. She waits for her loud mouth, bold and brash sister, who was more like her extroverted twin, even though they were two years apart.

"Hey, JoJo."

It is not Vaughn's voice that greets her. Jolene opens her eyes. It is Tanya. "Hey, T," Jolene says.

A warm smile creeps across her face. Jolene knows Tanya forced Vaughn to stay put in the living room while she came to find out if their sister was okay. Though Tanya was the youngest, she was the scrappiest amongst all of them. The first one to get into a fight over her sisters, or jump into a fight with her sisters. As the youngest, she was automatically able to get away with more than Jolene or Vaughn when they were children. She was the one they put forward to explain why the three of them had done something. They knew if Tanya said it, they would only get yelled at instead of whipped with their father's thick black belt.

Tanya sits at the table across from Jolene, and reaches for her hand. They clasp each other by the fingers and just sit in the energy. Jolene always called or visited Vaughn when she wanted to have a good time, a good laugh, and a good drink. Tanya was her call when she needed that quiet fierceness that exuded from her soul. With Tanya, it was the experience, the time spent, that doesn't require a conversation. Tanya is able to see her in a way few people do. In a way that is unencumbered and without demands. Around Tanya, Jolene can just be. She doesn't have to do anything, she doesn't have to pretend for anyone, she doesn't have to please or meet anyone else's expectations. She can sit and be herself and that is good enough for the both of them.

"How did the appointment go?" Tanya asks

"It was interesting?" Jolene says.

"What was so interesting about your first round of chemo?"

"That first shot through the IV your whole body gets warm and tingly. Like sex tingly, but only a little different."

"Different enough that you don't come in your clothes in the doctor's office?"

"Almost, but not quite."

"Jolene!"

"You asked. I told the nurse if the feeling didn't pass, I was going to have to leave and go home and find Mo and come back."

Tanya laughs. "You so nasty."

"Nah. I was just trying to get through the appointment. It's like when people know you're sick. They know something is wrong with you, they automatically treat you differently. They're extra nice to you, going out of their way to make sure you're accommodated."

"It's called caring about you," Tanya says.

"Not if it's forced. Y'all know good and damn well Granny Mae would not be sitting in her wheelchair in her Sunday wig, if she didn't know I was sick. She'd be right there in that back bedroom, fussin' and cussin' at Mama and Daddy because she still don't want to be in they house."

"Yes," Tanya begins. "But she loves you and she cares about you. She wanted to show up for you. We all did."

"I appreciate it."

"No you don't."

"You're right, I don't. It feels forced. But I'm supposed to act like I do."

"That's the truth," Tanya says. "But even if you act as stank as you feel, nobody's gonna tell you nothing because you're going through this."

"You can say it, T."

"No, I can't."

"Yes, you can. It's one word. Two syllables. It's not hard. Cancer. Say it."

"No."

"Say it, T."

"No."

"Say it."

"Why, Jolene? Why do you want me to say you have that?"

"So you're ready, T."

"Ready for what?" Tanya asks.

"You know what I'm talking about," Jolene says.

"I'm definitely not saying that. And if that's what you think, then you don't need to say it either. You're not leaving us. You're not going anywhere. You're going to win. You're going to beat this."

"Tanya, it's just me and you in here," Jolene says, holding Tanya's hand more tightly. "I have stage four aggressive breast cancer. I know you looked up what that means, just like Mo looked it up, just like Vaughn looked it up, just like Mama and Daddy looked it up, and then told Granny Mae. If y'all saw the same thing I saw, read the same things I read, you know I have thirteen months. Max. If I even have that left. I think that's what made the appointment so interesting."

"Why's that?"

"I was sitting in the chair flipping through a book of wedding floral arrangements while getting a treatment that may not work. I'm planning a vow renewal I may not even be alive for, thinking whether Mosiah would marry another black woman, or get a white woman when I'm gone."

"Jo, you can't think like that," Tanya says.

Jolene sees the tears fall from Tanya's eyes as she exposes the truth no one wants to accept. It is the reason she wanted to go home. The reason she didn't want to be bothered with anyone unless she absolutely had to. She didn't want to see the look in their eyes that Tanya has. She didn't want to see their sympathy, she didn't want their pity, or their niceties if that's not who they usually were toward her. She knew when she walked in the door and saw Granny Mae, dressed and ready like she was going somewhere, that they were all looking at her to see if they could see the death coursing through the inside of her body. They were looking at her to see if she was becoming a translucent skeleton, like the little boy in Lydia's favorite movie. They wanted to see if she was walking between both worlds; the land of the living and the land of the dead, waiting to be fully accepted by one or the other.

"You gotta believe you're going to get better, Jo," Tanya says.

"I know what I'm supposed to believe, but I know the reality too."

"And what reality is that?"

The question comes from her father. Jolene and Tanya look up to see their dad, solemn and somber-faced, waiting on Jolene for an answer.

"Daddy, I didn't see you come in."

"No, you didn't," Raenard says. "What reality are you talking about?"

"The fact I'm staring death in the face everyday when I look in the mirror."

"Are you still breathing?" Raenard asks.

"Yes," Jolene says.

"Can you still see?"

"Yes."

"Can you still walk, talk, smell, hear?"

"Yes."

"Then you don't look like no corpse to me."

"Daddy, you know what I mean."

"No, I don't. You said you staring death in the face everyday you look in the mirror, but from where I'm standing, you look pretty alive to me."

"I know I'm alive . . ."

"Then act like it."

"You got a little boy and a little girl and a whole room full of people out there waiting to see about you and you in here hiding."

"Can I be by myself for a minute, Daddy? Damn."

"You've been by yourself all day. You told Mo you didn't want him to come. You told your Mama, you didn't want us there. You told your sisters the same thing. You pushed us all away and we the people you need. We the people that's gon' help you get through this, and you got us at arms length like we not supposed to care. You can't do everything by yourself and you don't have to go through this alone."

"But, Daddy, I'm the only one in the house with breast cancer. So no matter what you say, I am going through this alone."

"No. You're choosing to go through this alone. You got a room full of people waiting to be there for you. But you do what you want to."

Jolene watches her father walk out of the kitchen as stealthily silent as he came in. Tanya releases her hand. She wipes her eyes and rubs her tearstained knuckles on her jeans under the table.

"C'mon, Jo," Tanya urges.

"Give me a minute," Jolene says.

She wipes her own eyes; the tears that welled up while her father scolded her for sulking. He wasn't a man of many words unless he was hurt or angry. When she got pregnant he lectured her every day. He ran scenarios on the outcomes of her life. Some were hopeful and optimistic, most others not so much. He demanded to know if she planned to just be a baby mama for the rest of her life, or if she planned to do something in spite of the circumstances of her swelling belly. Back then when she tried to hide herself away, cloister herself in the room she shared with Vaughn, in her bed, under the covers, he demanded that she get up, and get out of the room and defy the odds, the future that even he predicted for her. Now he's demanding her to do the same thing again. He's waiting for her to come out of the kitchen, to come out of hiding, to stand in front of her family and defy the odds, the mortal future they've all looked up, read about, whispered about, and wondered about to everyone but her.

It's a lot easier to face the world when you're giving life, then it is when you know yours is being taken away.

"C'mon, Jo." Tanya says pulling Jolene away from her thoughts.

"I'm coming," Jolene says.

She blows air out of her nose, wipes her eyes, and stands up from the table. "Let's go," she says.

Tanya takes Jolene's hand and leads her out of the kitchen and into the living room where everyone is gathered. Vaughn and her parents sit on the couch with Lydia laid over all three of their laps. Mosiah and Toussaint occupy the love seat, and Granny Mae's wheelchair is pushed in the space between both.

"Look who I found," Tanya says.

"It's about time you brought your butt out the kitchen," Granny Mae says without turning around. "You got people sitting out here waiting on you and you don't even speak."

"Hey, Granny," Jolene says.

"Don't nobody want your sorry ass "heys" now. You shoulda said that when you hit the door."

"Granny, I'm sorry."

Jolene walks over to stand beside her wheelchair. She kneels down and wraps her arms around her and squeezes her tight.

"Let go of me, lil' girl," Granny Mae demands.

"Nope. Not until you accept my apology."

"I'll accept your apology when you bring me that masters degree you been promising me."

"I'm almost done, Granny. I just have one more semester left."

"I thought you were going to take a semester off," Mosiah says from the couch.

"I never said that," Jolene says.

"I just assumed . . ."

"That's what you get for assuming, boy," Granny Mae scolds. "Jolene promised me a diploma and two degrees. I plan to collect. I got two, I'm waiting on the third."

"She needs to focus on getting better," Mosiah says. "She can take a semester off and come back to it after the treatment is over."

"She can. But for what? Chemo ain't goin' to affect her mind. She can think and get better at the same time."

"She needs to rest."

"Boy, don't you have her planning a new wedding for y'all? Talking about she need to rest, knowing good and well wedding planning is the most stressful thing in the world."

"How about you two not fight over me and about me, like I'm not standing right here," Jolene says. "I can finish this semester, and plan the vow renewal, and get chemo, and think happy thoughts, and whatever the hell else everybody in here wants me to do for them."

"Mom, can we go?" Toussaint asks standing up.

Jolene smiles at him as he walks to the front door, thankful for his petulant rescue. "Yes. C'mon, Lydia, let's go."

"So you're just going to leave?" Louise asks from the couch.

"Yes, Mama. I've had a long day. I told Mosiah when we left Mayo all I wanted to do was go home."

"Well, are you coming to church on Sunday?"

"As long as I feel up to it, I am."

"Good, because the pastor is going to do a special blessing over you."

"Really, Mama? The whole church knows."

"They just want to pray for you, Jolene. I know you not turning down free favors from God."

"No, Mama. I'm turning down free favors from you. I don't need anybody else in my business or looking at me crazy the way y'all looked at me when I walked in here. Let's go, Lydia."

"Mommy, why Nana want to pray for you for?" Lydia asks.

"She's just doing what she thinks is best," Jolene says. "Now let's go."

"Well, at least let us walk you to the door," Vaughn says.

"Y'all don't walk me to the door no other time I come over here. Why y'all being different today? I walked in here by myself, I can walk out by myself. C'mon, Lydia."

"I'm coming, Mommy."

"See ya, Granny," Jolene says half-heartedly.

"See y'all later," Mosiah says, raising a hand.

Jolene walks to the door where Toussaint waits for her. He opens it up and holds it until she is outside. For the moment it is just the two of them. He walks beside her as they go down the stone steps to the SUV.

"Thank you," Jolene says.

"You're welcome," Toussaint says.

The locks on the SUV click. Jolene turns around to see Mosiah, carrying Lydia, coming down the stairs. Toussaint opens the back door and gets in. Jolene waits for Mosiah. He puts Lydia in her booster seat and closes the door, brushes past Jolene, and gets in on the driver's side.

Well damn.

Jolene walks around to the passenger side and get's in. Mosiah is silent. He starts the engine and pulls away from the curb. He is quiet as the scenery changes around him, as he drives away from the quiet residential street to one of the busy thoroughfares of their Arlington neighborhood. He speeds through traffic on Rogero Road toward Fort Caroline, his mind racing the whole way.

She barely wants to plan the vow renewal, but she can finish a masters she doesn't even need? She can keep dishing out money for these damn credit hours, but is worried about how we're going to pay for her treatment.

"So are you just going to drive mad the whole way home, or are you going to tell me why you felt the need to get in a pissing contest with my grandmother?" Jolene asks.

"Jolene, you find every excuse in the book to not redo our vows, but you can finish school to keep doing the same thing you've been doing since you graduated the first time."

"I made a promise, Mo."

"You made a promise to me too."

"And I just said I'm going to do both, or didn't you hear that part when you were trying to think of a good response to win an argument with Granny Mae."

"How are you going to do both, Jolene? How?"

"The same way I've been doing everything else," Jolene says. "I feel fine right now. If every session is like this, I just might have something to look forward to."

"Why would you say that?"

"Because it's the truth. But nobody wants to hear that. They want me to say what I don't feel to make them feel better. I don't have any comfort to give, when I can't even comfort myself."

"Alright, Jo," Mosiah says, turning down Fort Caroline Road.

What did you expect?

He asks the question inside his mind. It plays over and over in his head as he zooms toward their enclave. The truth is not far behind it. The truth that he didn't know what to expect. He didn't know how to react when Jolene insisted he stay away from her first appointment, that he carry on his normal Wednesday activities as if their lives weren't changing every moment she was tucked away in a hospital room, attached to a machine pumping her body with a chemical substance that would kill all the good and all the bad inside of her.

"Don't put it in the garage," Jolene says when Mosiah turns down their block.

"Why not?"

"I'm going to go for a drive."

"For what?" Mosiah asks.

"Because I want to."

"Fine, Jo. Fine."

Mosiah gets out of the car and pulls Lydia from the back seat. Toussaint gets out behind Jolene. They close their doors and they are face to face. Jolene sees in him herself and Jemarcus. She sees the genes that made the intuitive teen, trying hard to be nonchalant, but deeply concerned. In him she sees that he knows, even though she didn't tell him. She is thankful for Mosiah's gift of gab, knowing she would not have had the strength to tell the baby she had when she was just a little older than he is now, the truth.

"You're going to be okay, Mom," Toussaint says.

"If you say I will, I will," Jolene says. "Go in the house. I'll be back in a little bit."

Jolene waits until Toussaint goes up the walk and into the house. When he closes the door, so does she. She makes a U-turn in the street and drives away from the house, away from the block of individual neighborhoods where the neighbors don't know each other, until she gets to the main road. Jolene drives until she gets to the highway, and drives the highway until she's circled the city three times. Not wanting to go home, Jolene drives with the radio on, the best song from every album making up the rotation on whichever format of station she flips to. She drives until she's left the highway and is sitting in a tree-lined lot where the lines are fading and families pass by her with blankets and picnic baskets to make an afternoon out of traversing the historic park on the banks of the St. Johns River.

With the engine running, the air conditioning blasting in her face, she slides her seat away from the accelerator and reclines it until it is touching Lydia's booster seat behind her. Jolene lays in the cool air of the dimming day and waits. She waits for her thoughts to recede, for the ideations bubbling at the front of her mind to dissipate, for the ruminations wanting to pour out of her to go away. They don't. Jolene rights the seat to a comfortable position. She reaches for her purse still on the floor of the passenger's side and grabs her journal. She opens to the page where she left off in the hospital, skips a line, and begins the new train of thought that won't leave her alone.

I just can't win for losing. It's like I try to do everything right. Get married, have kids, don't have babies out of wedlock. Well almost everything right. Then somewhere between doing everything right, here comes the bullshit of life. Why do I even bother? I should have just fucked around like everybody else. But that wouldn't have been fair to Mo. But would it have been fair to me, considering the circumstances? It doesn't even matter now with this bullshit cancer. The big C. The big sick. Whatever cute ass, commercial ass, trivialized ass name they have for it to make you seem like life doesn't suck, and you're not about to die. I wish they would say "fuck that" on them damn commercials and just call it what it is, a death sentence. People are living with AIDS now, but we're still dying by the bucketload from cancer. Maybe cancer needs a gay face. Or a straight face. Or a black face. Where the hell is Magic Johnson when you need him to get some shit and live to provide hope for the shit you're living with. Who do the cancer people get as a mascot, John fucking Mccain. He got the cancer Ted Kennedy had. I guess I'll see them both on the other side soon enough. And that's the fucked up part about all of this. They're old white men. I'm a young, black, woman.
Fuck this.
Fuck it all.

Jolene drops the pen and the journal into the passenger seat. She reclines and allows the tears that started to flow in the presence of Tanya finally escape full force. She wails as the air blows over her body, and her head begins to ache from the thoughts she can't shake because of the uncertain future only she will have to face.

God, where are you now?

Her mother comes to her mind telling her to make sure she is in church on Sunday so that she can be prayed over. Jolene sucks her teeth as she cries, despising the ritual that will be performed over her, already disdaining the pouring of the blessed oil, and the adding of her name to the sick and shut in list. She cries decrying all the ways that she will be treated because of the disease. The thin prayers that will be offered up in her honor, the moans of "Fix it Jesus," that will erupt throughout the congregation, and the pastor's sing-song message that will call for healing, but for God's will to be done; the message that will rely on a myriad of scriptures that will basically tell her God may want her to live, or God may want her to die, but either way, it is God's best because He doesn't make mistakes.

God is wishy-washy. I need the miracles of the Old Testament not that, now you see me, now you don't, of the New Testament.

Jolene cries until the vision in her mind changes and her mother's face is replaced by Toussaint. She sees the golden brown boy, with sleepy eyes, and heavy lips telling her, "You're going to be okay, Mom." She holds on to this vision. She holds on to this memory. It propels her to sit up in the car, slide her seat forward, and turn the ignition. Jolene holds on to the face of her firstborn and the tone of his voice as she leaves the parking lot for home. She puts all of the hopes everyone else has urged her to have for herself into him, and makes him the beacon for her heart to keep beating and her body to get better. Jolene sees Toussaint as she drives until his face warps into Mosiah. Warm, understanding, frustrated, brooding, moody Mosiah. She holds their dueling visages in her mind's eye, knowing they will be her strength when all of her own is gone. Not God, not her parents, not her sister, not her grandmother, not even her own daughter. She sees Toussaint and Mosiah. The one who said she will be okay, just because he believes it, and the one needing her to be okay so they can get back to the business of being themselves.

She sighs.

I can do it for them.

19.

They surround her in the bathroom. Toussaint, Lydia, and Mosiah stand around Jolene as she sits on a black stool facing the mirror, tufts of hair in her hand. Mosiah is behind her with his clippers. She promised herself that when her hair began to fall out, she would shave her head entirely, instead of prolonging the slow diminishing of her womanhood. She vowed she would detach herself from the feelings connected to the strands growing from her scalp. The hair she stopped relaxing in the name of health, even though she consistently wore it flat ironed straight with 410 degrees of titanium plate heat. She gave her word to herself that she would get rid of her crown and glory, even though it framed her face and hid her fat, because she would always be able to grow it out once she was well. Before Mosiah agreed to cut it he made her promise that the same meticulous care she put into her hours long wash day routine, would be the same care and caution she would put into her health, even if that required more faith than action.

"You ready?" Mosiah asks.

"As ready as I'm ever going to be," Jolene says.

"Mommy, can I sit in your lap?" Lydia asks.

"You're going to get hair all over you."

"I wanna sit on your lap," she whines.

"C'mon, Baby," Jolene says.

Lydia walks around from where she stands by Mosiah and climbs up on Jolene. Mosiah can see her wince with pain in the mirror, even though she doesn't emit a sound.

"Lydia, sit still," he snaps.

"I'm am," Lydia says.

"I got her," Jolene says.

"Mommy," Lydia says looking up. "Why you cutting your hair?"

"Remember what Mommy and Daddy told you," Jolene says. "Mommy is sick."

"Yes, but you said you were taking medicine."

"Good girl, you remember. Mommy is taking medicine, but remember what I told you?"

"Yes."

"What's that?"

"The medicine makes your hair fall out."

"Right. And what else did Mommy tell you?"

"That when you get better your hair will grow back."

"Exactly. Now are you going to sit still while Daddy cuts Mommy's hair?"

"Yes," Lydia says softly.

"Toussaint, hold my hand please," Jolene asks.

Mosiah waits until Toussaint has shifted over to take hold of Jolene's hand before he puts the clippers to her scalp. She buries her face in Lydia's thick hair as she feels the teeth of the clippers against her scalp. Mosiah starts along the side closest to her right ear. In one stroke her long hair pulls easily away from her head, revealing more caramel colored skin. Mosiah works front to back in trained rows until thick clumps, and long wayward strands, float to the floor around them. Mosiah goes over Jolene's head twice until all that's left is a light peach fuzz.

"I'm done, Jo," Mosiah says, squeezing her shoulder.

Jolene looks up from Lydia's hair and stares at her reflection in the mirror. She looks at her new self with old eyes. She examines her face like never before. With her hair gone and her head bald, she can feel the slightest of sensations in the atmosphere around her.

I don't know why bald chicks say this feels like freedom. I feel more naked now with my clothes on, then I've ever felt with my clothes off.

Jolene runs her hand over the top of her head. Feeling the rough stubble that remains and wonders when it to will shed and leave her with a dome ready to be shined. She sees herself for who she is without the safety and security of her hair. The weight she's beginning to lose is evident in her cheeks and chin from the strict diet she's been put on. The diet that consist of only whole grains, fruits, and vegetables. Foods that come prepackaged, nearly ready to eat, because the doctor's can't afford her picking up an erroneous bug from something fresh. Jolene sees her sunken eyes yearning for the sleep she's not getting at night because her body is too uncomfortable, too rigid in it's response to the chemo therapy, that it leaves her feeling tortured and fatigued, but unable to find rest when she closes her eyes. She stares at her reflection as her family tries hard not to stare at her. Everyone but Lydia. Her four-year-old looks on with mesmerized concern at her mother's solemn response to her new do. Cognizant of the little eyes following her every move, Jolene limits her reaction. She rubs her scalp, touches her face, and wipes her eyes to make sure the tears she's crying on the inside never fall on the outside. Lydia tentatively reaches her hand up in front of Jolene's face. She reads the look in her daughter's eyes and lowers her head. Lydia's soft palm caresses Jolene's bare skin, followed by small fingers exploring the scalp that's lost its covering.

Lydia brings her hands down and says, "Do you like it, Mommy?"

"Do you like it?" Jolene asks.

"You look beautiful," Mosiah answers.

Jolene nods. Toussaint squeezes her hand he has yet to let go. She squeezes his back and releases him. Bringing both hands to her face, Jolene covers her eyes and wipes away tears threatening to fall.

"Toussaint, open the cabinet and get that package on top of my hair products in the back."

"I don't see it," Toussaint says, opening the cabinet.

"That's because you have to bend down and look, lazy boy."

"The thing in brown?"

"Yes," Jolene says. "Take that out of there and hand it to me."

"Give this to Mom," Toussaint says, passing the package to Lydia behind him.

"Here, Mommy," Lydia says.

"Thank you," Jolene says.

"What's in there?" Mosiah asks.

"You'll see."

Jolene rips open the package and pulls out three tightly wrapped and folded pieces of colorful fabric. She tears the online store label off of one of the wrapped fabrics and shakes it loose, extending the pink and gold African print material with beige and brown accents, until her arms are stretched to their full length. Jolene shakes the fabric once more and then throws it behind her bald head. She starts wrapping the fabric like it's a normal scarf, tying a knot in the front. She then begins to bend, tuck, and knot the long pieces until she's made the fabric bloom into a flower atop her head. Jolene assesses her handy work she learned from a tutorial on the website where she found the head wraps. Looking from her own face, to those around her, she sees the immediate shift in reaction by Lydia, Toussaint, and Mosiah. She knows before they were being kind in their assessment of her appearance, now she can see the truth, that while she may be beautiful, having something adorning her head makes her more so.

"Where'd you get those?" Mosiah asks, breaking the silence.

"I bought them online from this website I kept seeing ads for."

"They're nice," he says.

"You look pretty, Mommy," Lydia says. "Can I wear one?"

"I'll have to buy you some," Jolene says. "What do you think, Toussaint?"

He looks at her closely before answering. His eyes travel over the intricate knots of the head wrap, to his mother's sunken cheeks and drooping eyes, knowing her hair did not hide the toll the sickness inside of her was taking on her outer body. He can still see the ravaging effects of the treatment they hope will cure the cancer. Toussaint looks at his mother's expectant face, the fabric atop her head adding artificial light and color to her complexion, and nods.

He says, "It's nice, Mom."

"Then that's all that matters," Jolene says, looking at him through the mirror. "I can jazz it up with some earrings and a necklace, and no one will know a thing."

"Sounds good, Jo," Mosiah says. "Sounds real good."

Jolene yawns in the mirror and stretches her arms wide behind her.

"Go on, y'all," Mosiah says. "Let your mama get some rest."

"Night night, Mommy," Lydia says.

"Good night, Baby. Good night, Toussaint."

"Go on, Jo, get in the bed," Mosiah urges. "I just have to clean up the clippers and the hair."

"No argument from me," Jolene says standing up.

She follows Toussaint and Lydia into the bedroom space. They walk out of the room, closing the door behind them as Jolene collapses on the comforter, not bothering to pull back the sheets, or toss the throw pillows on the floor. The pillow top mattress easily receives her body, even though it provides her aching bones no relief. Another side effect of chemo, of treatment, of the medicine that provides the closest shot she has to a cure.

Jolene lays on the bed, with her new printed wrap still affixed to her head. It is the royal appendage she bought, molded and shaped into her new crown until her glory grows back. She lets her fingers run back and forth across the down cover, enjoying the sensation of the fabric against her skin. Touching everyday things as if they were new or held some secret, is her new obsession. Instead of obsessing over her own death, she now, instead, chooses to focus on the minutia in life, appreciating every facet of every thing she comes across, the pedantic details right down to the cross stitching in the bedspread she lays on.

It's weird to think about how much I'd miss this stuff when I'm not here, even though I won't know what I'm missing.

The thought is fleeting as Jolene rolls over and gives in to the haggard look she saw in the mirror. She closes her eyes and waits for sleep to subsume her. She waits to be enveloped in REM that will set her adrift to dream dreams she won't remember when she wakes up. Arms folded beneath her head, Jolene lays there, listening to her breaths until she is no longer alone.

Still awake, she is keenly aware Mosiah is standing in front of her. She rolls again and gives him space to lay down. He adds his weight to the bed. Jolene sinks into the feel of the mattress. She winces in silence, used to everything hurting her, adapted to the pangs she can't shake, the ones she was told go with the territory of recovery.

Mosiah throws an arm lightly across Jolene's body. He drapes it across her blue sleeveless tank top, and the thin material of the shorts that have no pockets and on her frame, look more like boy shorts to wear beneath clothing, than actual clothing to wear outside of the house. His fingers flirt with the hem of her shorts that ride around the cheeks of her ass. She buries her face in her arms to hide the contortion of her features. She tolerates his touch, knowing it's been four weeks since they've connected. Four weeks since they've re-consummated their marriage and recommitted in body to their union. Mosiah cut her hair in jeans sans shirt. He gathers Jolene to his bare chest and let's his fingers play up and down the skin of her forearms until she stops him.

Jolene grabs his hand mid-movement, and sets it down on the bed. She does not wriggle out of his grasp, nor does she force him to loosen his grip around her shrinking mid-section, she only stops his continuous, incessant, strumming of her body in places where the skin is thin, and the bones are taught and rigid from the treatment that by day three of week four, can only be described as torture.

"I can't, Mo," Jolene says. "I want to, but I can't."

Mosiah removes his arm from around Jolene and rolls on to his back. He sighs his frustration at his unrequited desire, and waits for his lust to deflate. It's the one thing they've been missing, even though everything else in their household has remained mostly unchanged.

She insists on doing everything for everybody, but can't do the one thing I need from her. I even asked the doctor and they said she was okay as long as she felt up to it. She can cook, clean, go to school, talk to her sisters, help out with Granny Mae, go to choir rehearsal and all the other stuff she fills her days with, but she can't do this.

"I'm sorry, Mo." Jolene says.

"It's alright," he says. "I'm used to it."

"What's that supposed to mean?" Jolene asks, pushing herself up on the bed.

"Nothing, Jo. Nothing."

"It sounds like it means something."

"It's nothing," Mosiah says getting up from the bed. "I just . . . I just miss you, that's all."

"I'm right here, Mo."

"I know. That's the problem."

"What are you talking about?"

"I'm talking about how I watch you do everything for everybody, be all things to all people except for me."

"Are you serious right now?"

"I'm not saying you don't have good reasons for shutting me out, Jo," Mosiah says, softening the tone of his words. "I'm just saying it's hard for me to accept being shut out when you walk around here and act like nothing is wrong."

"I'm just doing what everybody wants me to do, Mo. What everybody needs me to do. I thought that at least with you, I could finally be honest about how I'm feeling, because you are the one person with whom I don't have to wear a mask."

"I guess I'm the lucky guy then, huh?" Mosiah sighs. "I get the short and shitty end of the stick, and that's supposed to be enough to get me through my days."

"I never said that," Jolene snaps. "I never said any of that."

"I didn't say you did, Jo. I'm just telling you how I feel. I miss you, that's all."

"And you think the best way to express how much you 'miss me' is to beat up on me and tell me how much you can't stand seeing me trying to keep myself together for everyone else. And the one person I trust to be vulnerable with, I don't offer the same courtesy, because I need him to be there for me instead of the other way around?"

"Jo, that's not what I mean."

"Well that's how it sounds."

"Like what?" Mosiah asks.

"Like you're blaming me."

"I'm not blaming you for anything."

He sits on the edge of the bed with his back to Jolene. He faces the doorway to the closet and the bathroom, and sighs again. "I'm not blaming you for anything. It's just hard to watch you go through this, pretending to be strong for everybody else."

"And that's where you come in, Mo. You're supposed to be strong for me right now, so I don't always have to."

"That's what I'm trying to do."

"Getting your dick wet is not being strong for me. And pouting because I physically, emotionally, and maybe even medically can't, isn't either."

"Jolene . . ."

"Don't Jolene me after you just blamed me for my cancer like I wanted this illness, this sickness reminding me all of the time of impending death. Don't you dare make me out to be like I'm a burden to you because I need you to be there for me, while I'm steady being there for everybody else."

"Jo, I'm not . . ."

She doesn't hear his protest, his plea for her to end her tirade. She says, "You know what you need to do. Wait. Wait 'til I get better. Wait 'til I get worse and die. Just wait. It'll all be over soon enough . . . one way or another."

Mosiah sighs. Officially turned off and shamed for no reason, he stands up from the bed and walks toward the door. He turns the handle, then turns around to look at Jolene. He doesn't tell her that her head wrap is askew, and her floral fabric arrangement is smashed so much, it no longer resembles the rose she made it into.

He says, "I miss being with you, Jo. There's nothing wrong with that."

"And there's nothing wrong with you waiting until we can be together again." She softens her voice, "I miss you, too, but there are other ways around this. Other ways I can be there for you and you can be there for me."

"Like what, Jo? Like what?"

"You didn't have to stop lying next to me. You didn't have to stop holding me," Jolene says, making space once again on the bed beside her.

"I guess not," Mosiah says.

He crosses the room in two strides and lays down next to where Jolene indicated. He gathers her into himself once more, and waits for her to settle. She winces but complies. Her hand is in his, their fingers intertwined, they lay together. Mosiah resists the urge to pull her any closer, to touch any part of her where she doesn't want to be touched. He holds her hand and settles for having her body beside him, even though he can't be inside of her.

"Thank you," she says, finally feeling sleepiness overtake her.

"Anytime," Mosiah says. "And thank you."

"For what?"

"For reminding me that just because you walk around here acting like you know how to do it all, it doesn't mean you don't need help.

"This is all the help I need," Jolene says.

"What's that?" Mosiah asks.

"You. Just you laying here next to me, for as long as possible, please."

Mosiah doesn't respond to her request out loud. He shifts his thoughts to focus from being needy to being needed. He lays beside Jolene, holding her hand, gripping her fingers, their hearts beating from their chests to their backs, thinking about the life they've made for each other, the comforts they've come to expect that are now totally upended, instead of gradually being pulled back, by something they could have never predicted or controlled. He lays there breathing with her, as she falls asleep first like she's always done with him, hoping, waiting and praying for normalcy to return to his life.

A song enters his mind and comes out in the hum of his lips. It is an old one he hasn't heard but will always remember, about the here and now. He hums to himself and Jolene's sleeping frame; the sweeping R&B ballad reminding him that in his here and now, his only job is to be the one faithful place where she can take off her mask, remove her crown, and be flawed and imperfect, naked and afraid, vulnerable and scared and still be all of his wife, and all of herself.

20.

It's Thanksgiving Day and where am I? Holed up in my bed too tired to move. At least this year I don't have to worry about eating too much and gaining more weight added on to what I need to lose. This year, I'll be lucky to keep down the macaroni, and I can't even have any greens. Mama refused to cook the ones out of the can and I can't eat the fresh ones; not in the bag, and I can forget about organic. Six rounds of chemo, radiation, and the cancer still isn't gone. Now the doctors are insisting on getting me into clinical trials and trying experimental treatments. I don't know who they think I look like, but I'm not their science project. You not gon' be poking and prodding on my body with a drug you don't know works, or a placebo that won't do nothing but waste the little bit of time I got left.

And if the doctors ain't in my face about something then it's Mo. I know he means well, but this wedding will be the death of me before the cancer. Every other day he's got a new idea, a new thing he wants me to pick, to order, to try. It helps a little bit, but I can only order so many flowers, browse so many look books, and watch so many bridal shows on TLC before I've had enough. We are already married, but he doesn't seem to get that.

Or maybe he does.
Maybe it's me.
Who am I kidding?
It's always been me.

If it was up to me we would have never gotten married the first time. We'd have just stayed friends with benefits, and maybe had Lydia. It seems like everybody getting married is getting divorced, while the couples who never marry seem to make it work. I don't know. I just don't know . . .

Jolene taps the top of the pen on the open page of her journal. She listens for noise in the house, but doesn't hear anything. Mosiah left with Lydia for his parents' house early in the morning. His parents and her parents, sisters, and even Granny Mae all agreed on what dishes to cook, and to then bring them back to her house for dinner later on in the afternoon. Jemarcus picked up Toussaint the night before to have dinner with his family.

They *always did eat early. The one time I went over there for the holidays when we were in high school, before I ruined their son's future, they had dinner at noon. At noon, my family is usually just putting the turkey in the oven.*

Jolene looks down at her journal page. She twirls the pen in her hand and sighs. It is the only sound in the house; her own breath, and it competes with the noise of the thoughts in her head. She writes:

Maybe immunotherapy or hormone therapy won't be so bad. Doctor Richards even said to try acupuncture. I'm still not a fan of needles, especially with as many times as they've poked me in the last few months. But if it helps. It helps.

Jolene looks across the bedspread to where her laptop sits closed. The paper she has yet to finish for one of her last classes, before she gets her masters, is still waiting for her somewhere in the recesses of the high tech notebook. She looks back down at the journal. The journal she picked up to procrastinate from writing her paper. The paper she should have completed last week when it was due, instead of asking for an extension since she's not working. A choice she's still not sure she's completely comfortable with.

Jolene reported for orientation in August just a few days after her third or fourth chemo treatment. The nauseousness had passed but the aches remained. By the end of the day, she refused to stand up from her desk. She couldn't bear the weight on her legs, ankles, even the soft pads of the bottom of her feet hurt.

Mr. Mackie, the other fifth grade teacher, made it his mission to tend to her, since his last teacher friend kept her word and left the school, the district, and the state.

"Why are you fussing over me now?" Jolene asked.

"Because you need my help," he said.

"Why do you always cling to people in trouble?"

"Because every time I help someone else, I'm also helping myself."

"How is that?"

"Don't you worry about that," Mr. Mackie said. "Let me handle it."

Jolene looked over the small teacher dressed in dark denim jeans, peanut butter loafers, and a short sleeved yellow button down with the logo of an open mouthed alligator in the corner of the pocket. She shook her head, mustered a smile and said, "Okay, Oliver Pope."

"Damn right," he answered. "I wear a white hat better than she ever did. And that's not easy to pull off with my pasty white ass."

"You stay pretty tanned though," Jolene said.

"Spray tanned. I figure it's the lesser of the evils to get the complexion I want, since I wasn't born with it like you."

"Be careful what you ask for," Jolene said.

"I'm not saying I want to be black . . ."

"Excuse me?"

"You know what I mean. Like I'm not fetishizing you. I'm just . . . I'm just trying not to be so pale without getting cancer."

Jolene didn't say anything back. Her silence was enough to trigger his apologies. He looked at her with his lips turned down and long sad eyes. She held up her hand and shook her head to stop him before he even began a profuse round of "I'm sorry's" and "I didn't mean to's."

"I'm okay, Mr. Mackie," she said. "I know you didn't mean it."

He slunk out of her classroom after she let him off the hook, but he didn't go far. Instead, he hovered outside her door, pacing back and forth between their rooms until Mosiah showed up. In that time, Jolene managed to get comfortable enough to lay her head on the desk between her arms, without disturbing her intricately tied white head wrap, and doze off. That was how Mosiah found her when he walked into her empty classroom, asleep on her desk. He took one look at her shrunken body, swallowed in her old clothes that were now at least one size too big if not two, and said to himself, *You're done.*

He gently massaged her bony shoulders through the thin fabric of her purple color block top until she awakened. The asymmetric cut of the top used to cling to her body from her shoulder, down all the curves of her waist, Spanx be damned. Now the stretchy fabric hangs away from her skin. Mosiah had to gather the shirt to her body as he rubbed her awake to make it stay in the place it used to hug naturally. He watched as she blinked the brief sleep out of her eyes and her focus sharpened to his steely gaze.

"You didn't have to come all the way over here to get me," Jolene said, once she could see him clearly.

"Looks like I did," Mosiah said. "How long has she been asleep?" he asked Mr. Mackie.

"About twenty minutes."

"Thanks, man," Mosiah said, nodding toward the teacher who was noticeably shorter than him. "Let's go."

Mosiah gathered Jolene to his chest, not caring if the layers of makeup she insisted on wearing to make herself look less sick, stained his crisp white polo with shades of brown and red. He held her around her waist as he helped her out of the school building. She allowed him to be her legs as she leaned on him for support. He was her mobility as they made their way through the halls and across the parking lot. Mosiah picked her up and put her inside his truck, fastened her seatbelt and then closed the door behind her. Jolene laid against the window frame, still cool from the blasting air conditioner she knew Mosiah liked to keep on the lowest setting, and the highest fan rate.

He got in beside her, closed the door, and pulled out of the lot without saying anything. Jolene relished in the silence and slept against the window. It wasn't until they had pulled up the driveway of their home, that he announced what was on his mind.

"Maybe you don't need to go back to work this school year."

"What do you mean?" she asked.

"You're getting chemo right now. Do you really think you need to be around a bunch of snot nosed kids, inhaling their germs."

"So I'm just supposed to sit home and rot away?"

"I'm not saying that at all, and you know it."

"Then what are you saying, Mo? What are you saying?"

"I'm saying you need to take care of yourself, first."

"I am taking care of myself. But it's not just me. We have a family, too, you know."

"I know we have a family. I got the family."

"And so do I."

"But you don't have to. You're sick. Whether you want to admit it or not, you're sick. Take the time they give you and then take some more, until you beat this thing and can go back."

"What if I don't beat it?" Jolene asked.

"You can't think like that, JoJo."

"Everybody keeps telling me don't think like that. Be positive. Don't be negative. See yourself cancer free. The truth of the matter is, I have stage four breast cancer. The worst kind, the worst one, all the worsts of the worsts, that's what I have. So excuse me if it's a little hard for me to see the roses blooming in the middle of the shitstorm."

Mosiah didn't respond. He snorted his frustrations. He didn't know how to craft the words to reach her where she was and bring her up to where he was looking from; the vantage point from which he saw their lives.

"I'm just saying take some time off," he finally said.

"Even if I take some time off from teaching, Mo, I'm still in school. I'm still a mother. And I'm still your wife."

"I keep telling you, I got us."

"Oh yeah? This from the same man who got mad at me because he couldn't have sex with me a few weeks ago?"

"Okay. I had a moment of weakness. I'm human."

"So am I."

"Jolene, you're going to run yourself into an early grave if you keep going the way you're going and not listening to anybody else."

"Did you ever stop to think that maybe what's keeping me going is everybody else I'm doing so much for, so I'm not focused on what's wrong with me?"

Mosiah shut down. She forced him to see things from her point of view, even if it was just a glimpse. However, he was stubborn in his resolve and recalcitrant in his response. He waited. Pulled down the mirror visor on his side and glanced at his face. He tipped his chin up in the air and looked at his beard he trimmed Monday when the shop was closed. He had found a gray hair. It shined brightly against the other near black hairs, adding character and age to what would otherwise be his youthful face. He plucked it with tweezers and flushed it down the toilet with the cotton pad he used to tone his skin, and ease the sensation after shaving his face. He didn't tell Jolene about the gray hair. He didn't give her time to notice it, he didn't want her to see the manifestation of his stress from his concerns about her. Mosiah examined himself in the mirror looking for more gray hairs, and measuring the layers of bags under his eyes, until he got tired of looking at himself. He silently closed the visor and turned toward Jolene, so that she would see he was as serious as she was stubborn.

He said, "You need to slow down. Take a leave of absence from work, take a semester off from school . . ."

"No," Jolene said.

"I'm not even done. What do you mean, no?"

"Just what I said. No. I'm not taking a semester off from school. I have two classes left."

"And you'll have two classes left when you go back too . . . after you're done with your treatment."

"No."

"Why?"

"Because."

"Why, Jolene?"

"You know why, Mo."

"No I don't, Jolene. What could possibly make you so adamant that you keep working and going to school, and doing everything else to kill yourself before the cancer does."

"Really?"

"I didn't mean it like that."

"Yes, you did."

"Well, if you think I meant it then answer the question."

"Granny Mae."

"Jolene, she doesn't need you to get a master's degree."

"Yes, she does."

"No, she doesn't. I guarantee you she doesn't even care."

"So what if she doesn't. I care."

"You're telling me you'll stop working, but keep going through your masters program?"

"I didn't say that."

"Humor me," Mosiah said.

"First answer this question, if I stop working and my family medical leave runs out, whose going to cover my insurance and my treatment at Mayo."

"Tricare."

"Is that even reliable with all the problems the VA has had?"

"You won't know until you try."

"I don't want to try and find out I can't get an appointment either."

"Then Medicaid, and you can switch to UF Health or Baptist."

Jolene sighed. It was now her turn to shut down. She leaned her head back against the cool window, closed her eyes, and thought about Mosiah's proposal. Leave work, finish school, and rest.

Isn't that what everyone wants. To not have to work if they don't have to. Isn't that the reason we all work anyway. To stop working.

Jolene thought about what her days would look like without having to beat the bell to work. In the pickup truck, beside Mosiah, she daydreamed about taking Lydia and Toussaint to school and picking them up. She daydreamed about finishing her last two classes at once and graduating in December from the online program, instead of in the spring. Jolene fantasized about the number of baths she would take in the clawfoot tub, since she didn't have to rush in and out by taking a shower.

This is the best thing to come out of this cancer diagnosis yet, she thought.

She turned to look at Mosiah and slowly shook her head yes.

"Okay," she said. "I'll take the leave."

"Good."

"Now who's going to get my car?"

"I'll have one of the guys from the shop go by and get it after we close up tonight. I've got to head over to the station and make sure everything is going right there."

"I thought you hired another crew to clean up the TV station."

"I thought about it, but it costs too much. The four of them can handle it. I just like to pop up on them and make sure they're doing what they're supposed to, the way they're supposed to do it. That's my name on their uniforms and on the contract. Gotta make sure it's right."

"Alright."

Mosiah leaned over and kissed Jolene on the side of her face. "I'll see you later."

Jolene mumbled a hasty goodbye and opened the door.

"Hold on," Mosiah said, scrambling to get out of the truck. "Let me help you get down."

"I got it," Jolene said.

She slowly maneuvered to the ground. Mosiah watched her as she walked toward the garage doors. He hit the button on the inside of his truck to let her go through the garage, instead of walking around to the back or front doors.

He watched until she had closed the door behind herself to go into the house. Jolene leaned against the door, staring out over the living and dining rooms, catching her breath, until she heard Mosiah back out of the driveway. Against the door, she looked over the house, and smiled to herself over all the time she was thankful to get back.

Laying in the bed, staring out over the closed laptop, and the journal of her unfiltered thoughts, still in her sweats she's taken to wearing as pajamas, she wishes she had something else to do besides wait for everyone to do things for her.

"Jolene, you sleep?" Mosiah yells, coming in the front door.

She doesn't answer him. She waits for him to come up the front stairs, tread down the hallway, and open the bedroom door to see for himself.

"No," she says as he pushes the door open.

"What are you doing?" he asks, sitting down on the bed.

"Wasting time. I should be writing my paper, but I don't feel like it."

"It's Thanksgiving. You shouldn't be writing papers no way."

"It's the only thing I *can* do since everybody else is cooking."

"You know you're thankful to not have to cook this year."

"I didn't say I wasn't thankful. I'm just bored."

"Tanya and Vaughn will be here soon enough to make you less bored."

"Yeah, but they're coming with everybody else."

"Well, what do you want to do until they get here, since writing your paper isn't happening?"

"I don't know. I would normally go to sleep, but I'm not tired."

"How about you pick a dress. It's the only thing you haven't done."

Everything always comes back to this damn wedding.

Jolene says, "To pick a dress, I have to try on a dress."

"No you don't. Not if you know your measurements," Mosiah answers quickly.

"How do you know that?"

"Vaughn told me."

"Of course she did."

Mosiah lays back on the bed and rolls over. He opens the laptop and rubs the mouse until it wakes up.

"Save my paper before you start opening and closing windows." Jolene says. She places her journal on the nightstand and then lays down beside Mosiah.

"You should've saved it when you finished."

"Save my paper, Mo." She smacks his arm with the back of her hand.

"Ow. I did."

Mosiah opens the internet browser and types "wedding dresses" into the search bar.

"What kind of gown do you want?" he asks.

"I don't know," Jolene says. "The one I tried on in the store with Vaughn was too small. And now I don't know what size I am."

"Well turn over and look."

Jolene rolls over in the bed as Mosiah hits the shopping tab on the search engine. She lays her head against his shoulder and watches as he scrolls through the images of brides, most of whom don't look like her.

"Type black bride," she says.

"I don't think you want a black dress," Mosiah says, once the search results come up.

"Yeah, that's a no. I don't need to look like Morticia. But that does give me an idea."

"Like what?" Mosiah asks.

"What if I don't wear white."

"So what color would you wear?"

"What about silver like Cynthia on *Real Housewives.*"

"Who?"

"Look it up?"

Mosiah types her request in the search bar and immediately comes face to face with the statuesque model in a flowing silver gown. He looks at Jolene and back to the pictures on the screen. Mosiah looks back and forth from his wife, who's now about the same size as the model though significantly shorter, and the retouched photos of the smiling, now divorced couple, and swaps out the heads in his mind. He sees Jolene in the one shoulder halter gown with the large bow, and nods his head and begins to hum.

"You like it?" Jolene asks.

"Do you like it?"

"I think so," she says. "I think so. Now we just gotta find a knockoff, because I know that dress ain't cheap."

"We'll find it."

"We?"

Mosiah nods and continues humming. Jolene rolls back on to her back as Mosiah serenades her with the daydreams of a soul legend who looked at her love blowing away. He closes the laptop and pushes it to the edge of the bed. Laying beside Jolene, he pulls her bald head to his chest as he transitions from humming to singing. The tenor of his voice and the alteration of the lyrics from he to she, envelop Jolene in a new musicality, markedly different from the strong soprano, and the easy falsetto of the original song.

"Thank you," she whispers into his chest.

He squeezes her shoulder and continues singing, "I want to be what she wants/When she wants it and whenever she needs it."

Jolene sings along in her head, trying her best to uninvite the thought that is always on her mind's periphery. It's no use. It charges forward and takes over as Mosiah begins the song again. He sings and she imagines herself, his love, blowing away, the fleeting and ephemeral wife overtaken by the fatal realities no one daydreams about.

21.

The spread on the expanded table is the concoction of ancestors imaginations. Mosiah, Tanya, and Vaughn worked together to add the middle piece to the dining room table to take it from seating six to seating eight adults. Mosiah then pulled out the card table from the garage and wiped it down for Lydia, Jovon, Riley, and Toussaint; since Jemarcus dropped him off as soon as dinner was over at his parents' house. And even then, between the two tables, there still wasn't enough room for all the platters of food. The smoked turkey sat in the middle of the holiday themed runner on the main table where the adults sat surrounded by several sides, competing for appetites. Jolene sat at one end of the table and Mosiah on the other end with both sets of their parents, and Tanya and Vaughn squeezed in. Granny Mae sat in her wheelchair with a TV tray in the living room, while all the kids were setup in the kitchen. Everyone's plates were empty, their belts and top buttons of their pants loosened, and toothpicks were in various states of withering to straw, depending upon how quickly each person had finished their food.

Light conversation has returned to both tables, but Jolene doesn't hear it. She doesn't so much ignore the cordialities between the Lewis' and the Walkers so much, as they arrive to her through a filter of water that decreases the volume of all words by a hefty percentage. It is the same for the brewing fight between the four children behind her. She doesn't ignore Lydia's whining for her brother and her cousins to stop teasing her so much, as she doesn't receive it the same as she normally would. She stares off into the space around her, her eyes darting around the first floor of the house she wishes was a lot bigger to accommodate the extra bodies now occupying her space. She looks out at the walls covered with age-progressive pictures of Toussaint and Lydia, prints of original artworks matted and hung in frames that cost more than the prints. With one hand propping up her chin, Jolene feels the sluggishness creeping up on her from her tryptophan infused feast. She adjusts the fit of her bold, red printed head wrap on her forehead, and makes sure the large bow is still winged to perfection.

"I love your head wraps, Jolene," Mosiah's mother says.

Jolene focuses on the woman across the table and smiles. She says, "Thank you, Ms. Pearl."

"Is that your only one or did you buy a lot?"

"I have a few?"

"Where'd you get them from?"

"I ordered them from an online store."

"You still do online shopping, even after all these hack attacks?" Louise asks.

"Yes, Mama."

"I do too," Vaughn says.

"What about you, Tanya?" Louise asks.

"Mama, if I can't get it online and delivered to the house, then I can't get it."

"I swear y'all the laziest generation of people I've ever met," Raenard says.

"Ain't that the truth," Paul says.

"Hold on, Pops," Mosiah says. "I may be a lot of things, but lazy hasn't ever been one of them."

"Oh, just throw us under the bus then, Mo," Vaughn says. "I see how you do. That's okay. I'm a remember that."

"Remember it," Mo says. "Write it down. Take a picture . . ."

"That's enough," Pearl says. "We don't need to finish quoting movie lines with bad words and all the kids in whistling distance."

"When did you see *Friday*, Mom?" Mosiah asks.

"It was on Netflix."

"Mom, Netflix doesn't just come on. You have to go to it and then search for it."

"What's your point, boy. I'm grown."

"Okay, Lady Pearl," Mosiah says.

"I wanted to know why all the kids kept sayin, "Bye, Felicia," and one of the young ones told me it came from a movie."

"I see," Mosiah says.

"Anyway, Jolene," Pearl says, rolling her eyes at Mosiah. "I like how you've been wearing your head wraps so people don't look at you like a cancer patient."

"That's what I am, Ms. Pearl," Jolene says.

She sighs dreading where the conversation may go next. As long as she's known Mosiah, she's known his parents, and she's always preferred his father to his mother, especially when they were kids. Now as adults, and married, they can't help but all be together at family gatherings, be it holidays or a week long summer reunion in the middle of a mosquito infested wilderness. Before Lydia was born, Jolene and Mosiah used to split holidays between her parents house and his, giving priority to whichever set of grandparents begged to see Toussaint the most. After Lydia, they did holidays at their own house and then stopped by the grandparents depending on how the day played out, but the reunions became non-negotiable. For Jolene, one week out of the year was a small sacrifice, but this year is different. This is the first time every member of the family has been in her space at once.

"I'm just saying you don't look like one, that's all," Pearl says. "Does she, Paul?"

"She looks like, Jolene, Pearl."

"Paul, you know what I'm talking about. I know you know what I'm talking about, because you do the sick and the shut in visits. You know how cancer patients look, especially when they lose their hair. They get all pale, and sallow skinned, and look jaundiced sometimes worse than newborn babies who haven't learned how to pee yet."

"Mama," Mosiah says.

"I'm just saying, she looks good," Pearl says turning to him.

At least it was a compliment.

"Thank you, Ms. Pearl."

Jolene bows her head and chuckles to herself at the woman in her short cut Sunday wig, and strand of fake pearls draping her neck. Ever since Jolene could remember, she'd always seen Ms. Pearl in fake pearls, shown off by a dress or blouse that always had a peter pan collar.

"You know some cancer patients just look like death walking," Pearl continues.

"Excuse me . . ."

"But not you, Jolene. You look good. You done lost some weight, face all chiseled, I can see your cheek bones. You look good."

"I guess cancer becomes me." Jolene snickers.

She glares at Vaughn who kicked her beneath the table.

"Just like that movie with Meryl Streep," Pearl says

"That's *Death Becomes Her*," Tanya says.

"How about we change the subject," Mosiah says.

"Anybody want dessert?" Tanya asks standing up.

"I'll take some sweet potato pie," Raenard answers.

"I got you, Daddy," Tanya says. "Anybody else?"

"Just bring both pies to the table," Vaughn says. "That way, if anybody wants some they can get some."

"How are you doing?" Vaughn asks, turning to Jolene.

"I'm in the fight of my life. How do you think I'm doing?"

"Is Mo, helping you?"

"Vaughn, you do realize I can hear you right?" Mosiah asks from his end of the table.

"I know you can hear me," Vaughn says, looking up toward him. "But I'm asking my sister if you're treating her right while she's sick."

"He does his best," Jolene answers honestly, looking at Mosiah. "Some things don't get done, but it's okay."

"Good," Vaughn says.

"You're just dead set on this damn wedding," Jolene says.

Mosiah smiles, even though she made a face at him. He says, "It's a vow renewal, not a wedding."

"Same difference." Jolene grins back.

At least she's starting to get into it, he thinks. Mosiah nods his head and sighs, relieved that she was at least a little excited about the ceremony, even if she's still frustrated about planning it.

"The best way to fight death and the enemy is with love," Paul says.

"C'mon, Reverend," Vaughn says in a whooping drawl.

"Vaughn, hush," Granny Mae says from the living room.

"Granny, I thought you were asleep."

"Because that's what I want you to think." Granny Mae Rolls from the living room to the edge of dining room table beside Mosiah. She says, "I done heard the whole conversation."

"Over the TV, Granny?" Tanya asks.

"Yeah, girl. That's how I knew to come over here and get me a piece of pie. Cut me a slice, will you, baby," she tells Mosiah.

"But, Granny, I was just getting ready for Reverend Paul here to give us a word on this here day of thanks," Vaughn says.

"Girl, stop playing with God before he strike all of us down," Granny Mae says.

"Well if we going to heaven, we may as well all go together," Paul says.

"I like the other word better," Vaughn says.

"The word is the word," Paul says. "It don't change. We all should be trying to get to heaven, and the best way to fight the enemy and death to get there, is through love."

"Amen," Pearl says.

"How is that?" Raenard asks.

The two men stare at each other. The reverend and the mathematician. The believer of the unseen and the believer in the tangible. While Raenard had never said he didn't believe, he never said he did either. When Jolene and Mosiah got married, it was the first time in years she actively remembered her father stepping foot into a sanctuary on his own free will. Jolene, Tanya, and Vaughn were raised in the church right beside their mother, as was Mosiah beside his own parents, Raenard on the other hand, took Sunday to sleep in, check the papers, and watch the game in his favorite recliner, with the sunken seat in the living room next to the old brown leather sofa. Jolene watched the men face-off at her dining room table wondering which way the latest iteration of their philosophical versus theological conversation would go.

Paul adjusts the top of his blue shirt, that was already unbuttoned, and clears his throat.

He says, "The bible says love is patient, love is kind, love is . . ."

"Love is everything we're not," Raenard interrupts.

"Which means it's everything we need, to get to where we want to be. Love is also a weapon."

"I guess," Jolene says.

"Why you roll your eyes?" Paul asks.

"Because, with all do respect, Reverend, I've read that verse so many times I can't even count. I've seen it framed in people's houses, and office buildings, I've even seen it on bumper stickers. And now there's a whole TV show about what love is."

"And?"

"And," Jolene continues. "Love is more than patient. Love is more than kind. Love is more than not envying or boasting or whatever else the apostle Paul said it is. You know what he didn't say about love . . ."

"What's that?" Paul asks.

"Love is rare," Jolene says loudly.

Mosiah stands up from his seat and walks around to where she is sitting. He pulls her close to him. She leans against his waist and cries the tears she didn't know had welled up and were ready to spill. Mosiah rubs the fabric of the head wrap at the back of her head, as she grabs his hand to make him stop. She pushes the head wrap away until it falls on her dirty plate. She only wears the head wraps for the benefit of others people, like Pearl, she dons the coverings to make acquaintances and strangers feel comfortable so that they don't know she is bald underneath. She cries and ignores the wrap black people who don't know her think she wears as an homage to her African roots she will never know, and others think she wears to express herself, or to act as her visual middle finger to the man. She cries while the fabric of her head wrap settles into the drying gravy and remnants of the dinner she ate without thanks. Against Mosiah's T-shirt, unwrapped and uncovered, she sheds tears with her vulnerability exposed the same way it is when she walks around the house unabashedly bald teaching Lydia to love herself as herself as she learns to do the same.

"What's wrong, Jo?" Mosiah whispers.

She cries in to him, coughing for air, hyperventilating for a clear passage for her words. Mosiah rocks her from side to side until she stops vibrating from the fears of her soul.

"I am shattered," Jolene says. "I'm trying to keep it all together, keep a smile on my face, keep going, keep doing, trying to be encouraged, and for what? What's the point?"

"So what would you rather do?" Granny Mae asks. "Die."

"Mama," Raenard says. "That's not nice."

"But it's true, Rae," Louise says. "You always did baby Jolene. Jolene you're not a baby. People live or they die. You got cancer. So what. Somebody else has it too. Stop wallowing in your feelings and recognize what's around you."

"Mama, that's harsh," Tanya says.

"And that's my point," Jolene says, pulling away from Mosiah. She wipes her teary, red eyes and says, "I keep putting myself back together again. After every appointment, every doctor's visit, every treatment, I'm still looking for the good news. I'm looking for the love that's supposed to get me through, and each time I think I'm good, that none of my cracks are showing, I break again. And the pieces get smaller, and it gets harder to get myself back together again. Do you know how hard it was to just get out of the bed this morning, get dressed, and look presentable just for dinner?"

"But, Jolene, you're not the only one going through it," Louise says. "Every day of this life is going to be hard, but you keep living."

"But what am I living for, Mama? Why do I keep putting myself together if in the end, I'm just living for a slow death, when all that will be left of me is the remnants of the woman, the wife, the mother, the teacher I once was. Just dust. Ashes to ashes, dust to dust, right, Reverend?"

"That's the enemy talking, Jolene.," Paul says quickly. "You've got to fight through that."

"With what?" Jolene asks. "Love?"

"Yes."

"Then I'm all out."

"No you're not. Look at you and Mosiah right now. He's standing there with you. That is love. Love is an action. It's a verb. Subject, verb object. I love you. That's your power. You have to do love, you have to put effort behind love, you have to exert love."

"See, I knew we were going to get a word on today," Vaughn says.

"Saying I love you doesn't mean anything," Paul continues. "It's not worth anything. You've got to want to see your love in action and at work for you. You've got to do love. Put your love to work for you and see how far it gets you."

"So far it's gotten me cancer," Jolene says.

"JoJo, you can't blame all the good or all the bad for where you're at right now," Raenard says. "Sometimes shit just happens. Excuse me, Reverend."

"No offense here," Paul says.

"It's like my husband was saying," Pearl begins. "Love is more than just saying I love you. Love is an identity you wear like armor. It's not just who you are or who you're in love with, it's also what you have right in your hand every day you're alive."

"I guess," Jolene says.

"You can't just be guessing, Jolene," Paul says. "You have to be confident. The bible says, 'Being confident in this that he who has . . .'"

". . . begun a good work in you will see it to completion until the day of Christ Jesus," Jolene finishes with Paul. "I know the word. I know the verses. We say the scriptures. Mo sings all the songs. Lydia writes me letters, and Toussaint will just come and sit and be around me. And I plan the wedding I don't even know I will be alive for. I keep having this dream that I'm planning a wedding for your next wife," Jolene says turning to Mosiah.

"There is no next wife. This is for you. Only for you."

"Jolene, you've got to imagine it, see it for yourself," Tanya urges. "It'll be good for you."

"See yourself in that dress you just picked out," Mosiah says.

"What dress?" Vaughn asks. "You didn't tell me you picked out a dress."

"The one Cynthia wore," Jolene says.

"From *Real Housewives*?"

"Yes."

"How're you going to afford that?"

"Just something similar to it," Jolene says.

"Why didn't you tell me?"

"Because everything ain't about you, Vaughn," Tanya says. "Damn."

"Since when?" Vaugn asks.

"Ugh, y'all get on my nerves," Jolene says.

"That's Vaughn," Tanya says.

"That's both of y'all," Louise snaps. "Just hush and listen to what your sister is saying."

"Thanks. Mama," Jolene says surprised.

Mosiah squeezes her body close to his again, trying to shield her from the speculative conversation she initiated taking on a form of it's own.

She looks up at him with dried tears and says, "I'm good."

"Are you sure?" he asks.

"Yeah. I'm good."

Mosiah walks away from where Jolene sits back to his side of the table. He wipes his own eyes as he goes to clear his face from any of his own tears that tried to fall. The liquid he can't play off as sweat, or spice from the food he's already digested.

Jolene looks out over the faces of her family waiting for her to say something to make them feel better. Each of them, with their own look of expectation, wait for her to say something with confidence that she will use their love for her as her armor, her weapon, her power to fight the cancer in her body that's been sullen in its response to the treatments concocted by man. She looks at them not wanting to disappoint them, not wanting to say that she drowned out their conversation, and stayed quiet through dinner because she couldn't help but think that this would be her last one. She doesn't tell them that she's been counting down the days and the months and has realized that unless the experimental treatments work, this is her last Thanksgiving, it will be her last Christmas, and by the time the date for their vow renewal rolls around, she may not be able to make it out of a hospital bed, or away from the hospice care she sees herself in. She doesn't tell them she may not even be able to wear the Cynthia inspired dress, and walk down the white runner covered, stone paved aisle of Casa Marina toward her husband who already is, standing in front of a gate that leads to the beach and the endless ocean.

She knows they are waiting for her to imagine the good things she does not see, the fortune and favor she was brought up to believe in, instead of the pragmatic reality of facts, figures, and medicine her doctors have been telling her with each dismal report on her progress.

She sighs.

I can always lie. I can always pretend. Just like when we were kids.

Tanya grabs Jolene's hand. She squeezes her palm and rubs her fingers across the back of her sister's frail, bony hand.

"I'm alright," Jolene reassures.

"That's not what I was going to say," Tanya says.

"Go ahead."

"I just want you to see yourself cancer free on your wedding day."

"Vow renewal."

"Same thing," Vaughn says, grabbing Jolene's other hand.

"Imagine it, JoJo," Tanya says. "Not for me, not for us, not for anybody else. See it for you."

"See it for you," Vaughn repeats.

See it for me.

22.

Jolene sees the sun flirting with the horizon. The dusty pinks, purples, and magentas of the seaside sky begin to break up the black of the night. The dark clouds break with spurts of white, as the luminous glow from the moon dims, and the stars are no longer visible against the onyx of the sky that's given way to shades of blue; navy and royal, yale, space and prussian. Jolene watches the colors of the sky change from the window of the heavy wooden door she is set to walk out of to meet Mosiah at the end of the aisle, beneath a white lattice garden arch. She sees the orange ball just breaking through the clouds. It clears the deep colors of the night in exchange for pastels. The baby pinks and blues at the top of the heavens are reminiscent of the balloons that waved outside the house when she had her baby shower while pregnant with Lydia.

Jolene watches as people file to their seats. Her parents, sisters, Granny Mae, Doctor Fisher, and a few friends are on the left. Mosiah's parents, and the men who work in his shop, and with him at the TV station, are on the right. Jolene sees a few young men's faces she doesn't recognize and knows they are the teens Mosiah told her about. The ones he was inadvertently mentoring, teaching them by proxy what it means to lead a life as a Black man.

She looks out over the sparse crowd and waits for the sun to get fuller in the sky. That is when Mosiah will walk out with Toussaint as his best man, by his side, for the second time. That will be Lydia's cue to walk out and throw the pink petaled roses on the white runner to make way for her mom.

The joyous atmosphere of their wedding do-over, disguised as a simple vow renewal, is a marked difference from the defeated despondence of Thanksgiving. Then Jolene didn't know if she would make it to this day, to a ceremony bathed in the new morning glory of the sun. But Doctor Richards gave her good news six weeks ago. In the same exam room where she was given a death sentence she was resurrected.

"Jolene, you're in remission," Doctor Richards said with a straight face.

Mosiah gasped at the news before Jolene had time to react. She watched Doctor Richards' face transform from dead pan to glowing smile. In the moment, she expelled all the breath in her body and inhaled reinvigorated life into her lungs. Without words, she brought her hands to her face and cried. In the exam room with Doctor Richards smiling and Mosiah at a loss for his own words, Jolene steepled her hands in front of her face as hot tears of gratitude ran down her gaunt cheeks. She wrapped her arms across her body, gripped her black sweatshirt, and rocked from side to side in the first real sign of thanks and praise she'd had in months.

Thank you, God.

She mumbled her thanks at first until the words of worship took over her whole voice. She repeated the devotion, getting louder and louder, finally believing in the God she doubted as she watched the numbers continuously decline on the scale, and her hair refuse to grow.

"Thank you," Jolene said, toward Doctor Fisher as she wiped her eyes.

"No need to thank me," she said. "You did all the work. I'm glad you decided to go into the trial. You've had amazing results."

"I am too," Jolene said. "But what's next?"

"What's next is you go back to living your life," Doctor Richards said. "Still be mindful of what you eat, and we'll see you here every three to six months, just to make sure your body is bouncing back from the treatment as it should and that the cancer is still in remission?"

"Can we travel?" Mosiah asked.

"I don't see why not, as long as you're careful," Doctor Richards said.

"Good," Mosiah answered.

"Anything else?"

"No," Jolene answered.

"Then I'll leave you two be. Congratulations, Mrs. Walker. You've come along way."

Doctor Richards left her chart on the counter in the exam room before walking out the door. Jolene watched as the door closed behind her. She stared at the knob waiting for it to turn, waiting for Doctor Richards to come back inside and say she'd made a mistake, that she had the wrong chart, that the cancer was not gone. Jolene stared and waited until Mosiah forced her out of her trance.

"What's going on in there?" He asked, touching the side of her head.

She hadn't even realized he'd gotten up and was standing beside her.

"I'm just waiting to see if it was a mistake," Jolene answered.

"It's not, Jo. You're cancer free. You're healed."

"I know. I thought it would feel different."

"What do you mean?" Mosiah asked.

"I'm grateful. I really am. And I'm shocked and surprised and all that, but now what?"

"Now you can send out those invitations you've been stalling on," Mosiah said.

"You're so pressed, like we're not already married."

"I'm always pressed when it comes to you. You should know that by now."

"I know," Jolene said.

Mosiah leaned in closer and kissed her temple. He let his lips linger against her head as she nestled against him, getting comfortable against the hairs of his face, and the fabric of his barber polo.

"You know what else we can do?" He whispered to her though they were the only ones in the room.

"What?" She asked.

"We can celebrate Valentine's Day," Mosiah said. "Consider it a prequel for the renewal."

Jolene smiles at the memory that led her to this moment as she backs away from the window overlooking her awaiting wedding party and guests. She looks down at her body wrapped in silver. Her reality TV inspired dress is only similar to the original in color and the initial cut. The thick strapped halter criss-crosses Jolene's neck in the front creating a sweetheart neckline. Beneath the gown she is solidly hooked into a push-up corset to fill out the front cut the dress. The ruched fabric wraps around the rest of her body hugging her slimmed out curves until it plumes in a fit of fabric, billowing out to the floor from her knees. Instead of a bow on her shoulder, Jolene wears a silver gele. The extra long fabric is tightly folded in rows at the front of her forehead and then fans out into a crowning halo. She reaches up to touch the pearl and rhinestone tipped pins that hold the fabric in place. Jolene picks up a mirror sitting on a small cart beside her, just inside the doorway, to look at her reflection.

The smoky eye makeup compliments the color scheme of her dress even though her eyelids are weighed down by thick false lashes blended into hers with several brush strokes of mascara. She tries to look past the makeup to the skin beneath the drag. She stares trying to see beyond the contour and highlighter, the bronzer and blush, to the woman inside. Her eyes travel the length of her face from chin to forehead and her fingers follow. They rest on the folded edge of the gele hiding the peach fuzz she dyed red beneath it.

No one has seen her hair since she dyed it the night before. Toussaint and Mosiah were staying at his parents house and Lydia was asleep in her bed. That's when Jolene ripped open the box dye and got to work turning the 1B brown peach fuzz of her returning natural hair into vibrant red. She printed and taped a screenshot of a nineties era pop star from to the corner of her mirror to inspire her while she worked.

Jolene looks in the mirror and smiles to herself knowing she will debut her freshly colored hair to Mosiah and her family during the brunch reception. Not even Tanya and Vaughn have seen her hair. She pinned and tied the gele herself learning from a slew of YouTube tutorials by Nigerian women. When her sisters walked into the bridal suite of the old inn she was wearing the gele, a thong, her robe, and jewelry. They fastened her in the corset and secured her in the dress. As far as they knew she would wear the gele for the entire day.

"Mrs. Walker, the sun is up," one of the attendants says walking up to Jolene.

"Lydia and I are ready," Jolene says. "I just have to wake her up. She wanted to take a nap since we had time."

Jolene walks toward the front of the restaurant to a table along the back wall of the building. Lydia is sitting in the chair her body prostrate over the tabletop. The basket of silk, artificial flowers she's supposed to throw is balanced on the edge, close to toppling. Jolene moves the basket to the center to keep from spilling the flowers and then gently shakes Lydia.

"C'mon, Baby, it's time to get up."

Jolene squeezes Lydia's shoulders and thighs and belly until she starts to squirm with wakefulness.

"C'mon, Baby. It's time for you to be the flower girl."

"I sleepy, Mommy," Lydia whines.

"You can go lay down with Mama and Granny Mae when you finish."

"But, Mommy, I tired."

"I thought you wanted to be the flower girl."

"I doooo."

"Then you have to get up," Jolene says. "Here, grab your basket."

"Mommy, pick me up."

"Hold on, Baby."

Jolene bends down and scoops her up and lays her on one of her bare shoulders. Then she picks up the basket with flowers and walks toward the back doors of the restaurant. She steers clear of the open path made for her and Lydia to walk down the aisle. She can see Mosiah and Toussaint waiting for her, as she skirts the door, while other people turn their heads waiting to get a glimpse of her.

"Ok, Baby, it's time," Jolene says, bending down to set Lydia on her feet. "Are you ready?"

"Yes, Mommy."

"Do you remember what you have to do?"

"Drop the flowers on the white carpet."

"Good girl. Let me look at you."

Jolene holds Lydia away from her body and examines her face. She wipes crud from the corners of her eyes and the bottom of her nose. Using her hands Jolene smooths the edges of Lydia's hair and fluffs her two pressed out ponytails.

"Okay you're all set," Jolene says standing up.

"Go now?" Lydia asks.

"Are we ready?" Jolene asks the attendant.

"Just waiting on you," she says.

"Go on, Baby." Jolene tells Lydia. "When you get to the end, go sit with Mama and Granny Mae."

"Yes, Mommy."

Lydia takes a step onto the runner and begins to walk. The acoustic song Jolene picked for her entrance plays. She closes her eyes and exhales as the soulful voice begins to sing about all that she is.

"It's your turn, Mrs. Walker," the attendant says.

Jolene opens her eyes to see the blonde haired attendant, dressed in all black, motioning for the attendant outside to tell the guests to stand. She steps on to the runner and blinks her eyes in the blazing sunlight of the new morning. Staring down the aisle to the end of the runner, Jolene sees Mosiah and Toussaint dressed in matching cream suits. Mosiah's skin is brilliant against the fabric, his hairline precise, and his goatee and beard neat. She looks from Mosiah to Toussaint, watching him fidget with his hands as he waits to be dismissed. Jolene keeps them both waiting as she waits for the music to move from the chorus to the bridge of the song with the lyrics that made her want to get married to Mosiah the first time around. She ignores the cell phones held up toward her face recording her every move.

"Now I stand before you with my heart in my hands," Jolene sings along in her head as she takes the first step down the aisle. *"I'm asking you to take me just the way that I am."*

Jolene walks kicking through the poof of her skirt placing one foot in front of the other to make her way toward Mosiah. She floats to where he stands. The sound of the ocean is constant behind them. The incessant crash of the waves drowns out the murmuring voices in front of them and forces them to focus on each other.

Mosiah is the focus Jolene has had since Doctor Richards told her she was in remission. The update didn't have the immediate effect she thought it would. Feeling too much at once after the words were spoken, fear and anxiety hung at the periphery of her body as she waited to be told that her good news was a cruel joke. Haunted for days Mosiah was patient with her. He took his time with her as he always had; attentive in their interaction and communication. Though he'd been working seven days straight for weeks, at one business or another, to make sure everything was paid for at the hospital and the renewal, he took a week off after she was given a clean bill of health to spend with her. As she worked through her own mixed emotions about being able to go back to work, and graduating with her masters, being able to eat normal foods, and spend more time with Lydia and Toussaint, she found the remnants of the girl she used to be with the best friend she could talk to about anything.

As if scales had fallen from her eyes, Jolene saw once again the Mosiah who visited her in the hospital after their junior prom because she had a baby at seventeen. She saw the boy she used to ride bikes and play tag with, the classmate she did homework with, the friend who carried her book bag when her belly was big, and the man who opened his life up to her and her son when he didn't have to. She saw all the things that made her fortunate that he had chosen her and reconciled them against her own internal war that she didn't deserve them. Following his lead, like a witness subtly instructed by a lawyer, Jolene found a balance between the passionate and companionate love she'd been jaded against by one bad experience. With every haircut he gave her, every time he helped bathe her, his sacrifice of his own needs, physical and emotional, she was able to bury the sprouting seeds of her bitterness, and revel in the love he'd always doled out that was magnanimous in its equanimity to eviscerate her discontent.

Focusing on his face now she sees what she intentionally blinded herself to under the guise of protecting herself from getting hurt again. Under the ruse that she was settling because she needed stability, and not because she was in love, Jolene spent the weeks after her positive prognosis with Doctor Fisher, finally unraveling the lies she chose to believe and taking off the armor she girded herself with just in case Mosiah ever gave her a reason to be ready for a "just in case."

With the ocean crashing behind them now and the officiant waiting to marry them again, she sees her "just in case" preparation was always unnecessary. She relaxes in her stance across from her husband ready to say "I do," without an inner plan ready to be activated if at any point in their lives he were to tell her "I don't," because she is confident enough now in their union to know it will never happen.

Mosiah grabs Jolene's hands. It is the first time he's touched her in two days. The first time he's seen her in the same length of time. His eyes cloud over, bathed in filmy tears of joy; happy to see her standing, dressed in silver, adorned with a sparkling crown, and holding on to his fingers with the slight curving grip of her own.

The water falls freely from his eyes as his father's voice rumbles behind them. Reverend Paul is cloaked in a black robe, with a white stole. His well worn soft leather bible, is jammed between his large hands. He grips it as he holds it pressed against his chest. He uses it to brace himself, or restrain himself, against the weight of his own body as he rocks back and forth from his heels to his toes calling out to the dearly beloved, and explaining why they are gathered together at the first light of morning.

"We are here to celebrate a love that hasn't gone cold," Reverend Paul says. "A love that hasn't grown stale or old. A love that hasn't succumb to the seven year itch. The love of Mosiah and Jolene."

The deep baritone rumbles of Paul's voice send shivers across Jolene's body. His voice combined with the cool ocean breeze of the March morning reveal goose pimples on her uncloaked arms. Innately in tune with herself, Jolene squeezes Mosiah's fingers working to wring the warmth from his palms into her own. She exhales and inclines her body toward the way of the rising sun waiting for the reverend to finish his introductions and give them their turn to speak.

"The good book says that he who finds a wife, finds a good thing and obtains favor from the Lord," Paul says. "Mosiah Alan Walker, you have found your good thing, the jewel in your crown worth far more than rubies. Do you take this woman, Jolene Marie Lewis Walker, once again, to continue to be your lawfully wedded wife, to have and to hold, for better or worse, for richer or poorer, in sickness and in health, until death do you part?"

"I do," Mosiah says.

Jolene watches him wipe the tears from his eyes as his dad begins his spiel for her as the wife. She listens to Paul while watching Mosiah's emotions overtake him. She watches him sniff back his feelings, and dab at the tears bubbling at the corners of his eyes, trying to catch them before they roll down his cheeks.

We've been through a lot. Most of it my fault. But he has always loved me.

Jolene sees Mosiah sniff one last time as he regains his composure. The trained Marine comes back into his body, taut and stoic, replacing the emotional man who is not afraid to wear his heart on his sleeve. She sees the man who convinced her to marry him years ago. The man who claimed her for his own when she hadn't even claimed herself. Beneath the cream suit, fresh haircut, and rented white shoes she sees the man who's always convinced her to lean toward the positive instead of toward the negative. The one who's always been able to bring her out of whatever funk she faced even if it was caused by him. The man who chose her and her son when he didn't have to, when he could have gone and enjoyed his prom, his life, his return home without the extra baggage and drama she brought along with her.

Choose joy.

The advice her mother and Doctor Fisher have been giving her for years comes back to her as quickly as the surf crashing against the sand.

I've finally got it.

She looks up into Mosiah's eyes as Paul asks her if she will again take Mosiah for all the good and all the bad for all the days of her life.

"I do," she says, looking into his old face with her new eyes.

Jolene holds up her hand for Paul to pause.

She says, "I do. Every day, I do. Every day, I choose you. You've taken my worse days and made them better for me and Toussaint. Even when you didn't have me you've always held me. You have worked and hustled your way to where we are to make us rich in spirit, and lacking nothing in our house. I have been sick and because of you, your persistence, your patience I am healthier than I've ever been. To you I owe you much more than thank you. I owe you an I'm sorry for ever doubting you. I owe you more than my love, but my life."

Mosiah stares at Jolene, gripping her fingers, bracing himself against her honesty.

Even though she's doubted me, she's come home.

He says, "Faith is the confidence in the things hoped for and the assurance of things not seen. Jolene. My Jolene. Seeing you here today in this dress and crown, looking as fine and as beautiful as you want to, I know my faith in you was for the right reason. Even when you didn't or don't see what I see, I still see you in all of your beauty, in all of your flaws, in all of your sickness, and thank God right now in all of your health. As long as you are mine, I am yours. I love you, JoJo."

Only the sound of the ocean is audible between them. They don't hear the whimpering sighs of their small group of guests, or see the subtle wipes of the eye from Paul behind them. Staring at each other, tears rolling freely down each of their faces they stare with the ocean at their back and its endless future for them marked in the time of the crashing waves. They barely hear Paul's sniffs and his direction to enjoin themselves to one another and reseal their covenant. It is only the awaiting eyes of the expectant, phone recording audience that instinctively moves them together. When their lips meet, their eyes close, their faces touch, and their tears mesh. Conjoined at the mouth they kiss to reaffirm their commitment to themselves and not just for the others watching.

Jolene and Mosiah kiss through the morning; as they take a new set of wedding pictures to add to the old set of memories. They kiss through the brunch reception prompted each time a glass clinks and by their own love lust that simmers between them waiting to be unleashed in the privacy of their suite.

They abscond from the courtyard reception as the revelry winds down leaving Lydia and Toussaint with either set of grandparents willing to take them. Inside their suite of the historic hotel music plays and Mosiah sings. He puts the emotion of the ceremony, of the exchanging of their vows, into the sweeping harmonies of the gospel drenched R&B melody vibrating in the background. Jolene stands in front of him as his fingers work unhooking the clasps at the back of her dress. He is methodical in his approach, focused to make sure every hook comes undone until the structured shape of the dress collapses into the trumpet plume already on the floor. He holds out his hand and Jolene steps out of the dress still wearing her heels, her garter in tact around her thigh, her gele still in place on her head, after she decided against revealing her color to everyone at once.

"One more layer," she says.

Mosiah turns her around again and works his fingers more quickly through the hooks of the push-up corset that kept her body and breasts in place in the dress. When he is done he unwraps it from her body and tosses it into the pile with her dress. He takes her hand and walks her away from the sitting area of the room and into the bedroom where the music is louder. Sitting on the edge of the beige, suede bed bench he turns Jolene around to face him. She towers over him in her heels. He pushes her body back slightly and drops to his knees. Her hands caress the top of his head as he presses his face to her leg and pulls down her garter with his teeth. He continues the tradition, usually done during the reception in front of the nosy eyes of many, in the safe sanctity of their suite overlooking the ocean.

Mosiah removes Jolene's strappy silver heels one by one, and the garter with them. He works his way back to the edge of the seat and pulls her closer. Looking at her body in pieces and parts he holds on to her hips and works the thin silver lace thong down the curves of her body until it drops to the floor and she steps out of it. Mosiah is drawn to her. He lays kisses on her stomach, starting with the line of life that never completely faded away after having two children. He kisses the fleshy folds that sag from being stretched, tattooed with marks that her body performed something miraculous. Mosiah kisses her source and then sits back on the bench to look at all of his wife. He stares at her new body. Gone are the ample curves given to her by excess weight. She is almost as svelte as her mother and sisters, but the stubborn thickness of her thighs, behind, and breasts remain in spite of the various treatments and eleventh hour trial she participated in to fight the disease.

Jolene steps toward Mosiah and reaches for his hand. She pulls him up so that he stands in front of her. Her fingers work on the buttons of his vest and then his shirt until she can push both off of his shoulders, down the length of his arms, and with a tug past his wrist until it drops to the floor. Her fingers work faster loosening his belt, unhooking the button clasp of his pants and tugging the zipper. The slacks fall without fight and Mosiah steps out of them and kicks the clothes to the side of the hardwood floor.

Now it is Jolene's turn to fall to her knees. She loops her fingers into the waistband of his boxer briefs and pulls them down, along with the tall length of his socks until he is as naked as she is. Mosiah pulls her back up until they are standing face to face. He steps toward her but she holds out her hand telling him to stop. He stays still in the tight space they've created between themselves in the large room. He watches as she takes her hand from his chest where she paused him and reaches it up to her own head. Jolene unpins the fabric held together at the nape of her neck and then pulls the gele off. She watches his eyes alight as he takes in the vibrant color of her hair.

"What do you think?" she asks.

Mosiah doesn't answer. He reaches his hand out to touch the curly coif shingled at the top of her head. She doesn't stop him. He pats the curls, gently feeling their softness and the layers of product she coated them with.

"When did you do this?" He asks.

"Last night after Lydia fell asleep."

Mosiah wipes the film of oil and gel coating the palm of his hand and the tips of his fingers along the side of his body.

Jolene asks again, "Do you like it?"

He brings both hands to the now chiseled cheeks of her face and kisses her lips. He pulls her toward him until he's backed up against the bench, his knees buckle and he's forced to sit down. Jolene rolls with the change in elevation and leans down to continue the kiss. Mosiah reaches his arm behind her back and pulls her even more toward him. She bends her knees on the bench around his thighs and sits in his lap. She can feel the heat between them, close but not connected, Mosiah holds Jolene where she is with both arms wrapped around her and kisses across her mouth, down the length of her neck to top of her sternum.

He lifts her lower body until he breaks her skin and the wet warmth he'd longed for, for months envelops him. He feels the shiver rattle down her spine. Her exhale against his ear is her own confession of longing. No longer are her aching bones, unexpected nausea, and feelings of despair keeping them apart. He is now her bedrock in another way. The cornerstone, connected to her source he holds her still astride him, his arms squeezing her back, her breasts pressed into his chest. He holds her tightly as she begins to rock.

Jolene initiates their rhythm with a steady sway in her hips. It is in time to the music he had long ago stopped hearing overwhelmed by the plate of sensory confection she offered him in the nude. She releases his thighs she had pressed together with her knees and allows her full weight to settle on him. Her roll moves from bottom to top as she undulates, forcing him to relinquish his grip and ride her waves until he finds his own power. He focuses on her body, running his hands up and down her sides, cupping her breasts, feeling nothing to cause him to wonder or worry.

Mosiah buries his face in her and kisses the skin of her bounty. He moistens her mounds, kissing, licking and sucking what's in front of him. Appreciating the feel of her against him he nibbles at her nipples until her rock of waves quicken. Mosiah metes out his pleasure until Jolene is the one wrapping her arms around his back. She squeezes his body against her, crushes his suckling head into her chest, and bounces her ass up and down on his body working to bring herself back from the edge of her own nirvana.

Mosiah gathers her knees into his thighs and stands up with her in his arms. He carries her to the side of the bed and gently lays her down atop the white hotel sheets, lowering his body to hers, he lifts his head, and reclaims her lips as he thrusts himself inside.

This is what I've been missing.

His thoughts are singular as he powers his way through the impulse, and the urge, to give in to his own body's wills and wants. He pitches and upshots his way through her love, sliding and gliding on her own pouring passion until Jolene claws at his shoulders and pulls at his face.

Her body movements beg him for more intensity. For punishing blows instead of sweet and fragile strokes. She pulls at him and bucks against him until he raises her legs up over his head and pounds into her center with precision strikes. Jolene meets him stroke for stroke until her knees are bent into her chest to keep her in place. Mosiah holds her down as he works out his own pent up frustration and fury, anxiety and optimism. He gives it all to her until he gives in to his own desires and explodes with the lava-like fire of his love. Jolene holds him in position as she comes to her own climax. The force of her own power pushes him away as she seeps with the satisfaction of their souls.

Mosiah collapses beside Jolene. He closes his eyes and turns his head away from the bright afternoon sun streaming in from the window of the room. He takes deep breaths to slow his heart as he pulls her into his body. She obliges scooting closer toward him as their senses for the world outside of their union come back to them. Another slow, bass heavy rhythm and blues love song comes over the powerful speakers from Mosiah's phone. He hums the consistent line of the distinct melody as she snuggles against his body. His arm wrapped around her frame, the notes of the music enveloping her, Jolene falls asleep with her fuzzy red head against his naked stomach. She drifts on the notes of the music coming from his lips and the sensation of feelings coursing through her body as if she was only dreaming.

23.

A dream. That is the only way Mosiah can describe the expanse of the white sand beach he walks on. It is nothing like the beach he left behind 36 hours ago where he said "I do" again. The see through blue sea is a stark contrast to the ocean he left. On the side of the shore where waves, further north, rip off and develop into storms churning the tortured souls of ancestors who could never be because they chose death over bondage, the water is all the shades of blue that could ever blue. Mosiah revels in its marked difference from the dirty, sediment filled water that crashes against the North Florida shore. The water he left behind is filled with the regrets and bad decisions of a people who conquered through human capitalism and then returned to the land they stole from to further their damage through imperialistic colonialism. Walking through the water on the Coast of Cape Town Mosiah is reminded there is more commonality between the black people separated by an ocean than there is a difference.

The hems of his white linen pants cling to his ankles coating them with ocean water and sand. His matching linen shirt is held together by a singular button. The ocean breeze makes the rest of the fabric billow about him, exposing his skin, taut and dewy with the drops of perspiration from the humidity heavy air and his own smug self-satisfaction.

The honeymoon Jolene could barely even imagine he made a reality. In the afterglow of their post-coital consignment to one another, Mosiah broke their spooned embrace to pad across their room in the old inn. Barley awake ,Jolene gingerly watched his movements thinking he was just going to the bathroom or turning up the air conditioning to clear the sweaty sex smell permeating the air around them. Instead he came back to the bed with a manila envelope.

"What's this?" she asked, sitting up beneath the sheet.
"Open it." Mosiah said.

Jolene took her time unfolding the clasp that sealed the envelope together, and pulling back the flap. She reached inside and pulled out several sheets of paper.

"What's this?" she asked again with her eyes scanning the pages.

"What does it say?"

"Are we . . . Going on a trip . . . To South Africa . . . Tomorrow?"

"We sure are," Mosiah said with a wide grin on his face exposing all of his teeth.

"But how?" Jolene asked, sitting up on her knees. "We're still paying for all the medical stuff. How can we afford this?"

Mosiah took the printed boarding passes from Jolene and put them back into the envelope.

He said, "You always say we don't go anywhere, we don't do anything, and we don't get anything new unless it's for the kids. Now we're doing this."

"How, Mo?"

"The insurance covered more than you thought, and the extra contracts I picked up to clean other buildings downtown came in handy. Instead of hiring another crew, I kept the four guys we had and just spread them out."

"You have been working like a dog," Jolene said.

"I know," Mosiah answered. "But it's worth it. Just to see that smile on your face."

Jolene pushed Mosiah on his back and wrapped her legs around his waist to thank him with another smile of her own. Her happiness and now the the feel of sand between his toes with the sun on his face, the breeze at his back, and the salt in his nostrils makes him forget what it took for him to arrive on the other side of the world.

He walks the beach to clear his mind of the hassle he had traveling. The four airports he visited in 36 hours each time getting the same question and giving the same answer. His frustration mounted as Jolene's impatience flared, both with him and the flight crews who acted as if she was not with him as he checked them in.

"Where is, Mrs. Walker," ticket attendants asked at every leg of the trip.

"She's sitting down," Mosiah explained.

"She needs to be here at the counter with you to check-in for the flight."

"I have her ID right here with me. You can see she's the same person. Only her hair is different."

"She still needs to be up here with you, sir, otherwise, I have to check you in as a single passenger and release her seat to someone on the standby list."

The outcome of these conversations were the same. Mosiah releases the anxiety they caused out toward the ocean as he meanders along the coast line in front of The Bay Hotel. He trudges the beach by himself while Jolene rests in their room. He prefers the surf and sand created by God to the man-made atmosphere surrounding the infinity pool that is the color of the ocean, and the wooden deck filled with white padded beach recliners and umbrella tents providing shade to the pale and pasty.

Mosiah finds a spot on the sand beneath a palm tree. He sits down and leans against the rough trunk of the tall palm providing little shade or comfort. He also sets down the journals Jolene gave him. On the flight she handed him two journals and an envelope. They were bound with twine and decorated with long purple flowers dotted with rhinestones, the unofficial color scheme of their vow renewal ceremony.

"Promise not to open them until we get there," Jolene told Mosiah on their flight from Johannesburg to Cape Town.

"Why not?" he asked.

"Because once you read them I want you to bury them."

"Why?" he asked.

"Because it's time for a new chapter in my life."

"What do you mean, Jo?"

She sat up from where she laid against the closed window shade of the plane and placed her hand atop her gift to Mosiah. At the bottom of the pile was the journal she took with her everywhere. The one that was either in the drawer of the nightstand or in her purse. The one that held her thoughts on everything, even the ones she was now too ashamed to share. It is the journal she wrote in about getting over Jemarcus, accepting Mosiah, her hesitation to marry, her consideration of divorce, and her displeasure over their often rushed pleasure. It is also where she poured out her gratitude that he didn't leave her when she realized how ungrateful she'd been, it holds her renewed point of view of the love they share, and what it's taken for her to find, choose, and keep her joy. The large, thick, train of thought, stream of consciousness journal she started writing in at the behest of Doctor Fisher after her staged intervention had never left her possession until she handed it over to him. She didn't finish the book but she was done writing in it.

On top of that was a thinner journal. This one filled with her prayers and affirmations. The prayers she prayed over Toussaint, Lydia, Mosiah and herself. It contained prayers written in pencil, and the resolutions to the ones that had been answered in ink; a visual cue of the permanence of God's will. That was at the front of the journal. At the back of the second journal were her affirmations. The ones Doctor Fisher suggested she say long before she took the advice. The affirmations that got her through chemo, radiation, and her reluctant participation in the clinical trial involving a mix of hormone and immunotherapy. The affirmations helped her get over the loss of her hair and the fear of the loss of her breasts. Written neatly in three columns over more than a dozen pages were the words, "choose joy" followed by the words, "I choose today," and other words of encouragement for the specific day.

The final piece of the gift Jolene wrapped and gave to Mosiah were two letters. Inside were her vows; both sets. The old worn paper of the vows she gave seven years prior, and the newly creased parchment she copied her impromptu vows and a few more thoughts from her heart onto. He did not know she had given him herself as his gift for their renewal ceremony. The parts of herself that she hid from him, that she often hid from herself outside of the lines of the pages she coated in ink. Outside of those pages she was the Jolene everyone needed her to be instead of the woman she was really feeling herself to be on any given day.

With her hand atop the gift of her old self Jolene looked at Mosiah on the plane, both of them dressed in their best travel sweats and said, "I can't make new memories if I keep holding on to old ones."

He said, "Sometimes it's good to go back to see how far you've come."

"If I keep looking back I'll never live in the present or move forward in the moment."

Mosiah didn't argue with Jolene on the plane. He nodded his understanding even though he didn't understand. He looked at her with the curly, fire red hair, clear skin, and determined eyes and accepted what she offered. He did not have a gift for her beyond the trip. He did not prepare a sentimental memento to mark the occasion, or a gift of his own gratitude that she'd said yes again. On the plane, in matching black joggers and sweat shirts he raised the arm rest that was still down between them and took her hand. He pulled her into him and squeezed her palm to feel the life pumping through her invigorating him. Inhaling her scent he closed his eyes and slept the last leg of their flight.

In the eye of his subconscious mind he saw her; the caramel coated, silver stunner, as she walked down the white runner aisle of the historic hotel toward him. He smelled her as she stood across from him; her body emanating with the scent of orange and brown sugar. She dazzled in the new sunlight of the day from her perfectly shaped gele crown, to the hugging dress against her body. Mosiah slept in a daze submitted to his memory of their recommitment and reconnection. The feel of her body against his. Her warmth, her wetness, her eagerness to please despite her need for release. He slept bathed in the recent anamnesis of their reconfirmed covenant. The thoughts calmed him through customs in South Africa and on the ride to the hotel.

Now facing the ocean on the other side of the world Mosiah buries his hands in the sand beside him and grips the grains with the same affectionate squeeze he gave to Jolene's hands every time they took off and landed on the plane. Her words are stacked beside them; the vows, the prayers, the affirmations, the inner workings of her mind that reveal the inner workings of her.

Mosiah picks up the biggest book of the gift he'd been given. The journal he saw her write in constantly. The one she always closed when he came in the room where she happened to be winding down. He opens to the page where the attached string bookmarks the place. It is neither the beginning nor the ending. It is not even the middle. He looks at the page written in her unrushed, oft practiced cursive scrawl and sees the date from more than ten months ago.

If I were honest, I'd be divorced right now.

"What the fuck."

The sentence disarms him and he knows it's supposed to. He knows she bookmarked the journal to a place where he would be directly affected by her words. He reads the sentence over and over trying to hear how it would sound coming out of her mouth instead of just streaming out of her pen.

If I were honest, I'd be divorced right now.

I guess she wanted me to see where she was to know how far she's come.

Mosiah rests against the uncomfortable palm tree and keeps reading. He consumes her self-doubt and subsumes her feelings of inadequacy. In page after page, from the recent past to the present, he peels back the layers of her psyche in her interactions with him, the kids, her parents, sisters, and students. He reads her words and sees her growth. The woman she was for the woman she is. The apparition of her old self shedding for who she was pruned and stretched into being.

Mosiah reads the words, leaning against the tree. The waves of high tide threaten to rise up until they crash against his feet. He stays put lost in this part of his wife, wishing he had something of his own to write. After every new entry he goes back and rereads the page she bookmarked for him. He reads the gut punching words that could have ended him if they had been acted upon, and then he moves on. He moves on to a later entry where he can see her change of heart and he wonders what made her see him differently.

He reads her words etched in black or blue ball point ink until his eyes blur and his head hurts. Mosiah closes the journal and sets it on the sand beside him. He picks up the envelope and opens the letters. He sees the worn, and tattered edges of the pages that were her first set of vows. The vows she wrote from disparate texts of scripture, used more as a tool to impress his mother and father who thought he was settling for less than he deserved, than shedding any light on her true feelings.

Choose joy.

That is the title line of the separate page of vows she said to him just two days ago.

He reads her words for all the reasons she's choosing him and will continue to choose him, again and again. A practice he knows she adopted from her mother because she wrote about it in the journal.

Mama said find a new reason everyday to keep choosing your husband. She sounded like she was full of shit when she said it, but at this point it doesn't hurt to try.

Mosiah initially chuckled at the sardonic line. Now he appreciates it more than the for little levity it brought him in the moment he decided not to wallow in the divorce that could have been, but instead revel in the celebration that was.

He reads through the second set of vows, some of which she said out loud before the small crowd, at their renewal. He reads the words until he has them memorized. He will add them as a half sleeve to his other arm. His first set of vows are permanently inked on the top half of his left arm. Markings she didn't notice until after their first round of coitus cleared the lust from her eyes and brought her clarity of vision to see the healing tattoo for what it really was and not just scars and scabs she thought never faded from childhood. He folds the paper of the second set of vows and places them in the breast pocket of his linen shirt for safe keeping until he can add them to his right arm.

Mosiah stands up with the journals and the vows from where he sits against the tree and walks toward the water's edge just inches in front of him. A set of feet with pretty painted silver toes stand next to him.

"What are you doing out here?" he asks.

"I was looking for you," Jolene says.

"I was reading your gift."

"I saw. I didn't want to disturb you. I thought you were . . . maybe . . . ready to come back to the room."

"I have to do something first," Mosiah says.

"What's that?"

"Set you free," he says, holding up the books and envelope.

"What do you mean?"

"Just what you said on the plane. If you keep looking back and comparing the future to the past you'll never move forward in the moment."

"Okay. And?"

"And, I'm going to let this part of your past, our past go, and I'm going to let you live in the moment."

"I already am," Jolene says.

"And I want you to stay there. I don't want anything else in the house that reminds you of where you were. You can remember without having a reminder."

Jolene nods at Mosiah. He stares at her trying to decipher what she's feeling that she's not saying. He looks at her in the long white sundress. The spaghetti straps offer no support to her slightly diminished breasts. The fabric floats away from her body in the wind picking up speed on the beach. Red hair, white dress, candy colored skin, orange and brown sugar scent, Mosiah overdoses in her essence beside him before turning back toward the water. He extends his hand toward her and she takes it. They take two more steps into the lapping surf. The water swirls around their ankles. The white caps bubble like soap suds, and then rush right back out on the strong current that has the power to kill no matter how calm it looks.

He bends down to a squat, hovering just above the water and sets the books on the sand. Jolene bends beside him, gathering the length of her skirt in her lap. He takes her hand and places it on top of the books she gave him as a gift, and then places his hand on top of hers. The surf comes back coating the bottom book in salty sea water. It runs out again. Mosïah holds their hands steady on top of books and envelope as the waves come back. They feel the power of the water wrenching to take what they hold. The book of prayers and affirmations is now wet. The water runs out. When it comes back again Mosiah lifts their hands. They watch the ocean overtake the envelope and pull the journals from where they had been pressed in the sand.

Mosiah and Jolene stand. The bottoms of their wet clothing swirl about them. They squeeze watery, salty palm, to watery, salty palm. On the beach, on the side of the world where their blood line originated, they watch as the books of inner thoughts, and the envelope of false promises and renewed commitments bobble away on the waves. They watch until they can no longer see the remnants of the records of what they'd lived through as told from just one point of view. They watch until they can no longer see the drifting of old memories. With the sun above them and the breadth of the ocean before them, Mosiah and Jolene turn back toward the hotel on the exotic coast. They walk toward the opulence and grandeur of their first real honey moon hand in hand, with one mind, and one heart aligned toward their future. Together, they walk away from the ocean and the unforgiving waves conquering their old selves and tired bodies renewed and ready to write a new story.

Coming August 2020

Beyond Bourbon Street

1.

"This is the type of shit I hate," Graigh says walking through the open french doors into the Bourbon Street hotel.

"And what's that?" Joy asks, dancing a two step behind her into the cool interior.

"All of this." Graigh waves her hand at the revelry. "The tourists, this ingratiating show for people who don't even get it."

"Graigh, it's Mardi Gras." Joy rolls her eyes. "All of this is for tourists. What's there to get? It's a party."

"Yeah, I guess." Graigh lags behind, letting Joy lead the way toward the bank of elevators that will take them to her floor.

Joy dances the entire way. Her body twists and shakes in time to the multitude of brass bands passing the hotel door celebrating the PG debauchery of Fat Tuesday in the daytime. Graigh watches her friend watching herself in the reflective metal of the elevator doors. Her hands shake rhythms into the ringlets of her long Indian temple curls. Her unrestrained A cups test the seams of her yellow tank top to see if they'll hold or let them spill out for the occasion. Her booty bounces up and down then sways into a rhythmic shake. Joy is the personification of carefree. Her light twerk denotes adulting in the daytime; belying the secrets yet to come when the sun goes down, and her husband returns to their room.

The elevator dings mid-shake. Joy continues her shimmy moving the rhythm from her ass to her shoulders. She steps onto the elevator inviting fellow guests to dance with her. An older beet red burned couple sidle up next to her toasted peanut butter arms and join her shimmy as they head into the chaos of the Mardi Gras parades.

"Graigh, what's wrong?" Joy asks half-heartedly, once the elevator doors close. Her bounce continues in the elevator thanks to the music piped in from the street.

"Nothing," Graigh answers, wrapping her arms across her belly.

"I know what it is," Joy says booty dancing in front of Graigh. "You're mad you can't drink."

"Oh really."

"Yeah. No one told you to get pregnant before carnival in the first place. Afterwards sure, but before? Who does that? You know you want a daiquiri."

"You have all the answers don't you?" Graigh says, stepping off the elevator onto the third floor.

"Of course I do." Joy walks the plush carpeted hall to her hotel door throwing her words behind her. "I mean you can't be mad at the tourists for enjoying the delectable offerings of the Big Easy. That would mean you're mad at me. I'm a tourist, and I'm your best friend, which means you can't possibly be mad at me. That's against the bestie code."

"What are we twelve?"

Joy ignores Graigh's flippant taunt and slips the room key out of the tight fitted back pocket of her cutoff denim shorts and inserts it into the door. The lock clicks and she sashays into the room letting her hips emphasize the long and short notes of the trumpets, trombones, and drums rocking the room walls from outside. The music moves Joy through the door, past the king sized bed, to the french doors leading to the balcony. Music blares from the street below. The plumage from colorful floats pass proudly carrying krewes along the route of the twenty-four hour party.

"I have to pee," Graigh yells to Joy on the balcony.

"Ok," Joy yells behind her. "Hey, Mista, throw me some beads."

A thick rope of colorful beads clatter on the wrought iron balcony railing. The clinking sound is muted by the resounding hush of the closed bathroom door.

Graigh unbuttons her jeans and eases them over her thighs. The rough hewn fabric stutters before following her fingers guidance to slouch around her ankles. She sits on the white hotel commode and exhales the tap water from her faucet. Looking at her almost flat belly she exhales again. Another kidney processed stream from the bottle of water she drank earlier whizzes into the pipe. She sits and drips dry, trying and failing to forget the uncomfortable truth. She is pregnant; twelve weeks pregnant with what she knows is not her first baby.

Toilet paper disintegrates against skin. She shivers as fingers brush against her super sensitive sex. Jumping makes the jeans comply over her legs and butt. They remain unbuttoned and barely zipped, a comfort for her mini pooch. She flushes the toilet and steps up to the immaculate bowl sink set in a granite counter. Her eyes avoid the large rectangular mirror hanging above.

Soap in hand, water running, Graigh scrubs her soiled fingers against the friction made suds. Her eyes nearly avoid contact with the mirror. Nearly, but curiosity wins. A raised brow. A lifted lid. One pupil gazes back at itself trying not to acknowledge the rest of the brown skinned face: the other tired eye, the narrow nose flaring just a bit around the outer nostrils preparing to spread with impending weight gain, bow shaped lips that refuse to disappear into a straight line no matter the height of her anger, razor sharp cheek bones cutting angles into her face, the one wrinkle line in her forehead with a small white head near her hairline, and the wispy hairs of her edges raising up from their shellacked gel prison to frizz in the humidity and heat with the rest of her fluffed, spiral curls. Thirty-eight and pregnant. Graigh shakes the excess water from her hands, rubs them dry on her pants, and succumbs to her reflection. It is the first time she has seen her unobscured self in weeks.

She glares at her belly from the raised hem of her blue tee. The thin pointed tips of three previously formed stretch mark lines peek from the band of her panties above the loosened waist of her jeans. The only physical evidence of what tried to grow. What tried to live. What tried to be born. What was stolen from her. Bushy eyebrows frown in the mirror. Graigh drops her shirt and turns away from herself. She walks through the cramped room with the oversized bed toward the brashy music beckoning from the balcony.

Joy sits in a high-backed iron chair, eyes closed, head bobbing to the music. Graigh silently takes the seat beside her and tries to imitate Joy's serene pose. Lids close over brown eyes, long lashes rest on the top of the thin skin covering her bony cheeks. Music encircles her, girding around her, putting a slight bop in her head and a tap in her feet. It is the exhale she's been waiting on all day. The one that alluded her in the bathroom as she sat with her thoughts trying to forget.

"And you're telling me you don't love this. You're a liar," Joy accuses, staring at her friend.

One eye opens with a menacing look but Graigh decides against her feeling to fight.

"It's not that I hate Mardi Gras. I love Mardi Gras. I think I just hate what Mardi Gras means in this city to people who aren't from here. It's just like everything else that people fly by here for; Essence Fest, Satchmo Fest, the Bayou Classic, Jazz Fest. It's an excuse to escape, celebrate the facade of good, and forget that there's still pain. Everybody wants to laugh, and joke, eat, sing and dance away their pain at the expense of someone else. I'm that someone else. The people that live here every day are the someone else."

"So you hate everything that your city is known for because tourists like me enjoy it?"

"Since you put yourself into the equation tell me how many times you've come to visit me in the last ten years? Twice. My wedding and now. Every time we talk it's 'Girl, I gotta come down there for Essence Fest. Girl, I gotta come down there for the Classic. Girl, I'm trying to be lit for Mardi Gras.' It's never 'Graigh I just want to check on you.'"

"Graigh, we are both married, with careers, and families. So yes I want to come see my bestie and get drunk and have a good time. That's not a crime. It's adulting. Besides you only come to see me when you're running from something. If it's not about drama then you don't even think about crossing ten to Tallahassee. So how about you stop trying to kill my vibe with your bitching and tell me what's really wrong with you."

"Well, let me tell you what else I hate first."

"What's that?"

"I love my home, but I hate the shucking and jiving. The trying to be trendy on TV. *Benjamin Button* was beautiful and *Treme* was necessary but *K-Ville* and *NCIS: New Orleans* seem to be over reaches. Performing for the sake of performing. People are only interested because of Katrina and that bitch is old, dead, and gone. Other people live here besides Brad Pitt, Wendell Pierce, and Wynton Marsalis. Jazz, food, and Hollywood's perception don't define us."

"What about *Queen Sugar*?" Joy asks.

"I'll have Ralph Angel's bail money ready anytime he needs it," Graigh says. "He is yummy. A whole meal."

"That's what I thought," Joy smirks.

"Don't judge me."

"But I am. So what does define you? Hating everything you just listed, with the exception of *Queen Sugar*, is like hating cheesesteaks and you're from Philly, or Harold's, Deep Dish, and Garret's popcorn in Chicago, or cayenne, chickory coffee, and beignets right here."

"Beignets make me nauseous."

"So is this a pregnancy rant or is this something you've been holding in for awhile?"

"It's not the hormones. People think because they know Bourbon street, been to one of Emeril's restaurants, and went on a ghost tour for Marie Leveau they know me. That they know us. Just because you can cook Food Network's version of cajun cuisine and texted money to the Red Cross after you saw *When the Levees Broke* doesn't mean you fucking know me," Graigh yells above the parade music.

"Who does?" Joy whispers.

"Hell if I know," Graigh whimpers. "I feel like I don't even know myself."

Tears cascade down her face as her quiet mulling drones to uneasy silence punctuated by symbols, and snare drums from the high school band marching in shiny polyester down the litter dirty street. Teenaged girls twirl batons and shake overly developed body parts. They strut in white boots and blue and glitter gold briefs past the hotel balcony to the next tourist stop along the parade route. Graigh watches the show below and blows a dejected sigh deeper than the attachment of life growing in her womb yet to protrude from her belly.

"Graigh, you are more than twerking and a second line," Joy says, offering her hand across the black iron table. "You are more than bounce music, Master P, Cash Money and Big Freedia. But when people have watched five seasons of *Treme* and all the other shit that shoots down here we believe we have a connection that makes us want to come down here, shake our ass, drink ourselves silly, and see the reality behind the mystery and the magic. We want to get to know you. *I* want to get to know you. In your element and not just the drama you bring to my doorstep."

Graigh accepts Joy's hand without acknowledging her own shortcomings as a friend. The gesture is their apology. The exchange of energy admits what they will never say in words. The touch clears the air for the truth.

Breaking the embrace, Graigh stands in time to see plumes of feathers pass by the hotel on the parade route. The masked Mardi Gras Indians bounce step and buck jump their way down the street following behind high schools; keeping traditions alive for the drunken foreign assembly who will never care to learn their roots.

"So are you going to tell me what's really wrong with you?" Joy asks, leaning over the balcony beside Graigh.

"I'm pregnant," Graigh says, looking blankly into the yet to dissipate crowd below.

"You are; twelve weeks pregnant. I know you've got your appointment tomorrow afternoon. I wished I'd known you were going to get knocked up when I bought these tickets. I'd have sent the Tonys home and stayed to go with you."

"I know."

"So how do you feel?"
"I'm scared shitless."
"And your baby daddy?"
"Who knows."

2.

"Halvert," the nurse calls from the doorway into the waiting room. "Elaine Halvert," she calls putting extra emphasis on the "T."

"Call me, Graigh. I go by my middle name," Graigh says, approaching the nurse.

"And it's Hal-Verr," Bombei says exaggerating the roll of his "R" as he stands with Graigh.

"Oh, I'm sorry, Dad. I just need mom right now," the nurse says, blocking Bombei's path. "We'll come get you when she goes back to see the doctor."

"Alright," Bombei says.

"I'll be fine," Graigh says behind the nurse.

The door shuts behind them and Graigh follows the nurse in lavender scrubs. Fabric swallows the legs and arms of the waif woman holding the clipboard. She leads the way to her cubicle motioning for Graigh to set her purse down on the cloth covered chair cushion beside the cluttered laminate desk.

"Take this in the bathroom there and give me a sample," the nurse says with a yawn. "Use these too."

Graigh takes the plastic cup and the packs of sanitary moist towelettes from the nurse's cold clammy hands to the sterile bathroom just behind the three rows of cubicles. Five other women in varying stages of pregnancy sit or stand around the other nurses in the office making documented small talk about the past month, or weeks, or days of their pregnancy. Graigh lingers in the bathroom doorway watching the women; some of the bigger ones stand with hands on their protruding belly, while others, apparently in the beginning of their birth journey, sit with their hands on clenched quads.

"Is there a problem, Mrs. Halvert?" the nurse says from her desk.

"No, I'm just catching my breath.

The bathroom door closes soundlessly. Graigh turns the small metal doorknob lock and leans against the white-gray door. Her eyes avoid the basic mirror hung above the sink. Against the door she breathes. Hands beneath her shirt, over the skin of her own belly, she pushes, prods and pokes at her pooch waiting for a flutter that doesn't come. A sigh emanates through her gut but expels like a normal breath. She pushes the sides of her work pants, already unzipped and unbuttoned over her hips to her ankles. The breathable wide leg fabric pools at her feet covering her pointed toe, red ballet flats.

Graigh fills the sample cup and sets it on a distressed, white-wood side table. She flushes, readjusts her clothes and washes her hands. When she is done, she carefully picks up her sample, walks slowly to the door and lets herself out into nurses' bullpen.

"Just set it on the mat, over there, under your doctor's name."

The nurse's abrupt instruction startles Graigh. She meets the woman's steely brown eyes that seem to stare through her and the door to the inside of the bathroom. Breaking the gaze, Graigh tips to the counter sharing the back wall with the bathroom and places her sample on the marked up puppy pad under her doctor's name. She is the only sample under her physician's name. Clicking heels mark Graigh's long strides and her return to her seated nurse. Lavender fabric is collapsed where the woman's belly should rest. The material folds in on itself, never meeting the bigger body that should be there.

"How are you doing?" the nurse asks loudly, undoing the velcro strap to take Graigh's blood pressure.

"I'm doing."

"You can answer better than that. Make a fist for me."

"I'm tired."

The nurse squeezes the pump to inflate the blood pressure band. Her eyes hawkishly watch the needle of the gauge. Graigh works to calm her rising anxiety from the standard test. She concentrates on her breath, making them even, slow, and and as deep as possible without coughing for air.

"Ninety over sixty-two. That's good. Have you taken any medication besides your prenatal vitamins since you were last here?" the nurse asks, picking up her clipboard.

"No."

"Have you noticed any changes in your body. Spotting, cramping, dizziness."

"No."

"Do you have any concerns you want to address with the doctor when you see her?"

"No."

The nurse finishes scribbling on the clipped chart and stands. Graigh does the same.

"Go on out to the waiting room and grab your husband. I'll come around from the other side and take you both to the exam room."

Flat heels click down the linoleum past the bay of nurses to the door from whence she came. Bombei stands as she enters the room. The uneven mix of mothers and the handful of fathers barely adjust their eyes as she glides around squared chairs and end tables to where he stands.

"Everything alright?" Bombei asks.

The long hairs of his full beard tickle her skin as he whispers against her forehead. His soft lips leave a kiss as he pulls her close. She doesn't answer his question, only nods her head affirmatively, that for now she is alright.

"Come on back," the nurse's voice calls from a door adjacent to the check in counter.

Bombei takes Graigh's hand and pulls her gently behind him toward the nurse. They follow her into the office's inner sanctum, around the corners of the maze like halls, until they reach an open door to an exam room.

"Come on in. Mom we want you to take off everything from the waist down. Dad you can sit here," the nurse gestures to a dusty, cracked leather stool by the room's large window. "When you're finished drape this across your waist. The doctor will be with you shortly."

Graigh waits until the wispy nurse closes the door tightly behind her before she slides her black slacks and lace panties down her body. The sable tunic top covers her behind in the cool air conditioned room.

"Can you hold these for me, please?" Graigh asks with an outstretched arm toward Bombei.

He takes her hastily folded pants and underwear and sets them in his lap while she hops up on the exam table. Her butt jiggles with the bounce. A tremor of feeling ripples from a dimple down the sculpted and toned sides of her hamstrings and calves. Sitting on the exam table, Graigh pulls the ends of her shirt up from under her butt and drapes the excess fabric around her hips. She pulls the paper covering the nurse handed her apart, gently peeling each corner until it is prostrate and laid against her legs. She does not look at Bombei. Her eyes filled with with warring emotions over her belly avoid his gaze. She finds his feet perched on the bottom rungs of the stool he placed directly in front of her as if he wanted to conduct the exam himself.

Silence settles uncomfortably around them. The tick of the small round wall clock is loud above the unspoken thoughts of husband and wife. The typical traffic noise of Canal street is nearly muted beneath them. It only asserts itself in the chortling rumble of a semi truck headed back to the highway. The rays of the February sun stream through the large window at Bombei's back, immediately radiating heat on his body. Small bubbles arise on his skin and slide to his jean belted waistband beneath his thin, gray knit shirt.

The heat from the sun will be his excuse for the same sweat bubbles forming on his forehead and beneath his armpits, though he knows the latter began the moment Graigh disappeared with the nurse. His unanswered question lingers. The answer necessary to salve his own nervous energy.

"It's Doctor Marcella," a lilting voice accompanies a knock. "Are we ready."

"Come in," Graigh calls hoarsely from the exam table.

She looks up from Bombei's feet for the first time as the doorknob turns. The doctor's white coat flutters as she steps inside the exam room, and swirls around her brown slacked legs as she presses the door closed with one hand. The loosened ends of her salt and pepper pin curls bounce around the crisply starched collar of her beige striped blouse folded on the outside of her lab coat.

"How are you guys doing today?" she asks, pushing the rolling stool between Graigh's clenched knees and Bombei's prayerful pose.

"Fine," Graigh mumbles.

"Put your feet in the stirrups, lay back, slide down, and open your knees. Any changes since I saw you last month? Any butterfly flutters?"

"Nothing. Not that I can tell," Graigh says, crooking one elbow over her head and placing a protective hand over her stomach beneath her shirt."

"That's normal. It's still early. You're only twelve weeks. Give me a deep breath. Okay a little pressure," Doctor Marcella says, inserting a lubed finger into Graigh's vagina to check her cervix.

"Release the breath."

Graigh exhales as Doctor Marcella removes her digit. She rolls to the hulking trash can and discards the white latex gloves. Standing she scrubs her hands wrist to fingertips over and over under the water from the sink and then dries her hands on rough brown paper towels.

"Now, we're going to get that baby's heartbeat and do an ultrasound to see how it's doing in there," Doctor Marcella says, turning around to face Graigh and Bombei. "Any ideas on what you're having yet. Boy or Girl."

"No," Graigh answers.

"Just healthy," Bombei says, lowering his praying hands from his mouth to speak.

"Well, you'll find out soon enough. This is going to be a little cold."

Doctor Marcella squeezes the ultrasound activator gel on Graigh's tummy pooch and moves the heart monitor wand around in the goop. Left to right, up and down, from her navel to her knickers, and hip to hip Doctor Marcella searches with a stern face, and keen ears until the steady drone of what sounds like "wow wow wow" emerges from Graigh's uterus into the room for the gathered trio to hear.

Graigh and Bombei exhale the breaths they'd been holding since they arrived at the patient tower of University Medical Center. Their audible relief tells more about how they'd really been feeling than any one word answer to contrived questions ever could.

"The heartbeat is strong. Let's take a look and see how your baby is doing in there."

Doctor Marcella turns on the monitor to the ultrasound machine. The dark screen comes alive in shades of black, white, and gray. Warm, world rough knuckles skim Graigh's belly, gliding the wand through the gel as the makings of a baby manifest on the screen.

Graigh stares at the large pronounced head and the oval body. A head, nose, mouth, torso and the makings of feet lay serenely on her uterine wall waiting for more genetic information to stretch and grow before birth.

"It's really there?"

The words escape her mouth breathily. They interrupt Bombei's prayer. His hands drop to his sides and feet touch the ground as he sits on the edge of his stool.

"That's my boy," Bombei says with a smile slowly piercing through his closed mouth.

"Or girl," Doctor Marcella says with a smile of her own.

"Just healthy," Graigh says, sliding her fingertips through the gel of her belly to where the wand lays projecting the image on the screen.

"It doesn't look like a graham cracker anymore."

"They grow fast," Doctor Marcella says. "In utero and in life. You two should cherish these moments."

Graigh presses gently along the places that seem to match up with the sonogram image feeling for her baby's head and body.

"Your baby is healthy. We just want to make sure you are as well," Doctor Marcella says, rolling away from Graigh. "How's your breathing?"

"Okay, if I'm moving slow," she answers, still looking at the screen feeling for where her baby is supposed to be.

"And if you're moving faster than slow?" Doctor Marcella asks, handing Graigh a damp and warm white towel. "Use this to wipe off the gel when you're ready."

"If I'm moving faster than slow my breaths are shorter, more measured, but not quite gasping," Graigh answers. She stares into the monitor, eyes fixed on the image of her baby, serenely sleeping waiting on God's first breath of life.

"I take it then you don't do much exercise."

"I walk," Graigh says turning her head. "We walk the neighborhoods. The ninth, Lakeview, the East, St. Charles Street, the Quarter, Treme."

"How is her breath when she's walking, Dad?"

"It's fine," Graigh answers, wiping the gel and losing the image of her baby.

"I asked Mr. Halvert."

"She does alright," Bombei answers. "If we walk longer than thirty minutes though, she talks to me less than usual. That let's me know she needs to slow down. But we're alright."

"I suggest both of you do some meditation and work on deep breathing. Or swimming. Try to increase your lung capacity. Especially you mom. You're going to need it for labor if you're planning for a natural birth. Yoga could help too."

"I guess," Graigh shrugs. "What would you like me to do with this?" she asks, holding the dirty towel away from her body.

Doctor Marcella takes the towel by the corner and drops it on the sink counter.

"We'll see you guys back in a month. That's when you'll find out if it's a boy or a girl; if you like. I'll leave your chart here. Take it to reception and they'll make your next appointment. Take care of yourselves. Both of you. Especially you mom. You gotta carry that baby.”

The doctor leaves as briskly as she came in. Her coat flutters behind her, walking shoes squeak on the linoleum as she travels down the labyrinthian hall to the next room where another patient waits.

“Feel better now?” Bombei asks, standing from his stool and handing Graigh her clothes.

“I never said I was upset.”

“No, you didn’t. And neither did I.”

“So why are you asking if I feel better?”

“Because I can tell you do compared to when we first arrived.”

“I could say the same about you.”

Graigh pulls the ends of her tunic over her unbuttoned and partially zipped pants. Clothes in place she snatches the chart from the counter, opens the room door and marches out. Bombei catches the closing door with his hand and follows behind his stalking wife to check out.

“We’ll see you back here in four weeks,” an older lady with a nasally voice and green-veined hands says as she hands Graigh an appointment card.

She shoves the card into her pants pocket and flings the door open on the waiting area. Out one door and opening another Graigh is face to face with her reedy nurse.

“Everything go well with Doctor Marcella?” she asks, seemingly more out of polite policy than actual concern.

“Yes. Nothing to worry about.”

“That’s good to here,” the nurse says with cloying warmth. “See y’all again soon,” she drawls.

The nurse waves with an Wednesday Addams smile. It is the only brightness to the woman with sunken eyes and cheeks in a uniform two sizes too big even if it is probably an extra small.

“Thank you,” Bombei says. “We’ll see you next month.”

He pushes the main door to the office open and waits for Graigh to pass through. She huffs by him, briskly walking down the hall and to the emergency exit door, opting instead for stairs than to wait for the elevator. Bombei too descends the steps in the dank, dust filled, musty stairwell until he reaches the ground floor where Graigh waits beneath fluorescent lighting just outside the doorway, hand on her belly, coughing, and catching her breath.

3.

"What's wrong?" Bombei asks, turning the music down on the car stereo.

"That's the third time you've asked me that and we haven't even left the parking lot," Graigh answers, looking out the window.

"The first two times I asked you didn't answer me."

"Nothing is wrong with me. We had a good appointment. I'm just tired."

"Ok, Graigh," Bombei sighs. "Take a nap. We'll be home in a little bit."

He gives her the room to think, and clear space in her mind for whatever thoughts are taking over. He's known this woman for nearly fourteen years, his wife for twelve going on thirteen, is moody and mercurial. She falls in and out of fits of gray just as her name suggests. Keenly aware she's in them, she chooses to brood, instead of talk, to retreat into herself, instead of opening up to the possibility that there are people who care enough about her to listen or help.

Bombei turns out of the parking lot of the massive University Medical Center complex and heads down Canal Street toward Claiborne. The sparsely leaved trees in front of the glass faced building cast shadows across the car in the late afternoon sun. At Claiborne Bombei waits at the light to turn left. A half full street car passes by them at the viaduct. Left over Mardi Gras revelers hang out of the windows of the electric train. Ropes of beads visible around their necks, and styrofoam cups filled with unfrozen drinks tells of a party still going despite the new season of lent. In the deeply Catholic city the site of the spring breakers, the sunburned and spritely aged hanging on to their youth, distinguish a marked difference from the folks on foot with black ashes crossed on their foreheads.

At the green light Bombei turns left on Claiborne opting for the scenic route home instead of the highway. He turns the radio back up. WWOZ. The city's lone jazz station.

He catches the middle of a brass band song, one he doesn't know off hand. He nods his head to the steady beat of the music, fingers working to keep time and tap the unfamiliar beat on top of the steering wheel.

The music plays as he leaves Canal Street, the gateway to the city's downtown, toward the Treme. Fingers tap as the track changes to Louis Armstrong's "What a Wonderful World." Satchmo's husky voice fills the sedan scratching through Graigh's armor as she harmonizes an alto hum with the legendary trumpeter. Looking out the window she watches the immediate and dramatic change of scenery from new, modern construction to historic, old, and rundown. The streets narrow. The roads get more bumpy; the potholes more deeply felt. The grass wild and unkempt takes over strips of concrete paths meant to be sidewalks, and spills over the curb into the street. At Robertson and Louisa Bombei speeds past the cemetery. The high walled fortress looks more like a prison than a resting place. It is the only oddity, but what has always been, in the neighborhood that appears recovered. The exact opposite of what they passed a block over when they were headed to the hospital. There cars congregated in a grassy field where a garage will never house the parked vehicles beside the shotgun home the drivers either came to visit or live.

Small boxy air conditioners hung outside of the green trimmed windows of a white paneled house. The paint dingy and peeling needed several coats just to sparkle, juxtaposed against a vacant purple home with the windows boarded up on the neighboring corner. A brick faced church, with a well manicured lawn behind a wrought iron fence, and another old white paneled building that was probably a corner store made up the four corners a block away. The latter also had white paint, dingy, peeling, faded and cracked covered in large graffiti, grass and vines. The corner is post-Katrina personified. Some moved home, some moved home and recovered what was possible and rebuilt what was necessary and some, many didn't come home at all. It is New

Orleans. One block of beauty, one block of normalcy, one block of poverty but every block of pride.

Bombei crosses the Industrial Canal slowing on the rickety bridge over the murky water that claimed hundreds of homes. He sees Graigh cross herself as he drives over the bridge. A habit she's had since he's known her. When they first began dating he asked her about the cross.

"Why do you always do that?" he chuckled in jest. "Praying the water doesn't come alive and swallow you whole?"

He thought the joke would break more of her ice, but he was met with a thicker berg than he guessed. She stared at him blankly, wide set eyes sliced to slits, lips parted but no smile forming.

"I pray for the souls who were swept away in the water without warning, for the families who survived but lost everything, and for God to forgive the city engineers, realtors and everybody else who thought it was a good idea to cut a canal and sell folks land on the other side of it, below the sea, because railroad tracks were no longer enough."

He didn't respond to her impassioned diatribe. No head nod of agreement, no apology for his insensitivity. He let her words sit heavy between them, storing them away to be analyzed another day; to use as a catalyst to pick her apart when she was willing. But in fourteen years she has never been willing. She is an open book with most of her pages stuck together.

The lower ninth ward greets them on the other side of the bridge. A community of it's own design where the waves are friendly, the food is good, and the poor Black charity case remains wanted for the crime of purporting stereotypes to desperate journalists without a second source of confirmation. They stop at the light at Claiborne and Caffin Avenue. The campus of Dr. King Charter School beside them. The red gated school where their child will inevitably attend from pre-k to twelfth grade buzzes with activity. Parent pick-up, members of the marching band playing random notes ahead of practice, and teens on corners talking trash to each other and into their phones. The sounds of youthful voices lift into the air and rustle through the thick foliage of old trees shrouding the school in shade. This so-called beacon of hope, that was here before, negates the neighborhood's unearned narrative. It's existence challenges the argument that to live and be black in the ninth, is to be ignorant and poor.

Bombei races past the new fire station and makes a left three blocks later onto Charbonnet. A house painted seafoam green and surrounded by a red fence sits on the corner blazing in the sun. It is the unofficial welcome mat to the block where empty spaces wait for their owners to come home. He pulls beside Graigh's old white pickup truck in the carport of their two story home. It's the sentry among their neighbors. The addition built on top of the original shotgun that was later squared off for more modern comforts.

"We're home," Bombei whispers above the stillness in the air.

Graigh groans awake, stretching her arms as high as they will go in the cars interior. Her jaw drops low into an elongated yawn as she arches her back and rolls her head on her neck bringing life into her stiff joints.

"I need a nap," she proclaims from the passenger seat.

"Go inside and lay down then. I've got to go back to work."

"Ok," Graigh says, reaching for the door handle.

"Wait, let me help you out."

Bombei jumps out of the running car and runs to Graigh's side. She stands in the space of the open car door. Eyes alight, her lips smirked, hands reversed on her hips, with her thumbs in the dimples of her back.

"I'm pregnant. Not handicapped. You can close the door."

It slams shut as she steps high on to the butter and beige tiled porch; restored to look like the original her grandmother picked out before she was ever an itch in her unknown daddy's pants. Graigh unlocks the white iron storm door and the heavy wooden door behind it. Still air greets her face at the threshold. Bombei stands close behind, the breath from his mouth curls circles of heat around her neck as she steps into the formal living room.

It is now as it was before the storm. White. White sofa, white love seat, white walls, mahogany and glass end tables and coffee table. Large rectangular mirrors sparkle in glittering, crystal frames. It is the room of reckoning. The room to sit in your Sunday clothes and take pictures on Christmas, Mother's Day, and Easter. It is the room of tribute and honor, a love letter to her grandmother that she wanted everyone to feel welcome in.

From the living room she passes into the dining room. The room that once shared space with an everyday family room is now home to a wood slab sanded down by Bombei's hand, and stained coffee black by her. It is one of the many projects they completed together, building projects that helped them build their relationship as they restored what she lost. The table set for twelve is empty save for a centerpiece of fresh fruit. It leads into the chef's kitchen. Where there was once a wall for a bedroom the space is now completely open. A wide butcher block island marks the separation point between the kitchen and dining room, with four black, leather backed bar stools on either side. The kitchen, back splashed in dove gray subway tiles, sparkles in the natural light from the French doors that break up the back wall of gray quartz countertops. The polished stainless steel appliances gleam in the rays. The rarely used recessed lights lining the ceiling remain as unnecessary as the rectangular tiered chandelier.

Graigh takes the stairs in the middle of the kitchen to the second floor. The stairs she demanded take the place of what used to be the home's only bathroom. Bombei fought her on the design. He wanted to keep the three piece washroom. The bathroom he suggested be designated for guests. He thought the rounded, spiral staircase was a bit much for the modest home even with the second floor addition; especially for the neighborhood. Graigh, was flippant in her compromise. "I got it, and I'm going to flaunt it." The construction of a half bath forced her to square off the stair case, but she got her way in the end because the transition from floor to floor still happened in the heart of the home.

Graigh is snuggled beneath a royal blue fleece blanket when Bombei gets to the loft at the top of the stairs. Her eyes are closed but he knows she's not asleep.

"I gotta get my horn so I can meet the kids at practice," he says.

"What are you practicing for, Mardi Gras was yesterday?" Graigh asks without opening her eyes.

"St. Joseph's Day," Bombei says, passing Graigh into their master bedroom.

He picks up his trumpet case and walks back into the loft. Graigh lays uncomfortably on her side, trying to get used to the position she will be forced to sleep in once her belly gets big. Normally a stomach sleeper, her legs are adjusted for the new position. One foot sits atop her leg, knee in the air making a perfect triangle. She lays posed, pretending, with the blanket up to her nose, bearding around her ears, her attempt to avoid conversation.

"What's wrong?"

"Why do you keep asking me that?"

"Because I haven't seen you like this in a long time?"

"Seen me like what? How am I today?"

"Just different. Quiet. Distant. Guarded."

"I don't know why you think that. We had a good appointment. We're through the first trimester. The baby is healthy. I'm healthy. We're working. The house is done. What could be wrong with me?"

Her question bothers him. Maybe because it's not a question at all. It is a statement, rhetorical, a period at the end instead of a question mark. It is her tone that tells him to leave. The upspeak. The inflection. She's baiting him, goading him into a disagreement he will regret. When she is angry her eyes smile and her words cut. Her tone is her warning, her dare.

"I don't know what could be wrong with you," he begins. "I know you're different. Ever since you found out you were pregnant, you've been different. You won't let me in, you won't let me help, you won't let me know how to get into you, or how to help you."

"Bombei, we've been together almost eleven years. If you don't know that by now, I don't know what else I can do to help you."

"Don't shut me out, Graigh, and make it like I'm the incompetent one. I know your past is rushing back at you. I can see it in that glazed, glass look you have."

"What are you talking…"

"You don't want to talk to me about it. Fine. But you need to talk to somebody. Especially before my baby gets here."

"Is that a threat?"

"It's not a threat. I would never threaten you, Graigh. It's a suggestion."

"One you've made repeatedly."

"Exactly. The record is broken, the stick is a twig, and the horse is dead. Talk to somebody. I haven't seen you this way since we met."

Bombei doesn't wait for her to respond. Trumpet case in hand he jogs down the stairs leaving Graigh behind in the same awkward position she argued from; closed eyes, knee in the air, blankets tucked around her frame. Disconnected.

He marches out of the kitchen, through the rustic dining room and to the door, avoiding the mirrors begging him to look at himself, to see the irritation, the frustration, and the defeat in his win. He had the last word, but he was no closer to what he wanted.

On the porch he descends the singular step to the paved walk way carved between two uneven loaves of St. Augustine grass. The grass is nothing like it was when he first saw it, when he first saw her. Standing in the spot where they met, the lawn lush and sumptuous, manicured and vibrant, he laments the marriage that has transformed into everything his home is not; unrefined, at the precipice of ruin and resurrection.

He crosses the grass to the carport, rounds the still running car, and gets in on the driver's side. The jazz instrumental blares as he backs into the pebble rough street. He turns the corner heading back toward the red gated school at the corner of Caffin Avenue. He drives toward his students leaving his past behind. Leaving behind the spot where he stopped when he first came home after the storm. The spot where she stood. The spot where they met about fourteen years ago.

Acknowledgements

We made it. Or I made it. Well, if you've followed my writing journey on social then we made it. Yeah, we made it, because even though writing is a solo effort, I definitely couldn't have done all of this alone.

Soooooo . . . First and foremost, thank you God for helping me get through another project with everything else going on in my life. A big thank you to my husband, to whom this book is dedicated, for being patient with me while I completed this project and several others.

Big thanks to my dynamic duo of an editing team Roy and Arvita Roberts-Glenn. You guys push me to go beyond the surface and leave everything on the page when it comes to these characters and my many others.

As always a big, big shout out to Gisette Gomez of Zodiac Studios for another dope book cover. From the newsroom to working together long distance you always manage to bring my vision for a cover to life. If anybody judges our books by their covers I know they'll walk away with intrigue that makes them want to know more.

This story is completely different from *Four Women* and *The Appeal of Ebony Jones* and I hope you, dear reader, enjoyed it. It was inspired in part by my husband and in part from a statistic I heard at work that says, "Black women aren't more likely to get breast cancer, but if they do, they are more likely to die from breast cancer." Upon hearing that my immediate question was, "Why?" Through Jolene and Mosiah I wanted to mine the details around that statistic and breast cancer in general, but I also wanted to tell a story of enduring love that can survive many ups and downs including internal self-doubt.

I want to say thank you to Dr. Saranya Chumsri from Mayo Clinic for giving me the nitty gritty on cancer treatments and the statistics surrounding black women and cancer. Thank you to Aretha Rodgers and Desiree Walker for sharing their experience as survivors. And last, but certainly never least, thank you to you for reading this novel and investing your time, energy, and money in this story. I don't take it for granted at all. So thank you, and look for more to come from me and NEW Reads Publications.

Peace,

Nikesha

About the Author

Nikesha Elise Williams is an Emmy award winning news producer and author. She was born and raised in Chicago, Illinois, and attended The Florida State University where she graduated with a B.S. in Communication: Mass Media Studies and Honors English Creative Writing. Nikesha's debut novel, *Four Women*, was awarded the 2018 Florida Authors and Publishers Association President's Award in the category of Adult Contemporary/Literary Fiction. *Four Women*, was also recognized by the National Association of Black Journalists as an Outstanding Literary Work. Nikesha lives in Jacksonville, Florida, but you can always find her online at www.newwrites.com, Facebook.com/NikeshaElise or @Nikesha_Elise on Twitter and Instagram.

www.ingramcontent.com/pod-product-compliance
Lightning Source LLC
Chambersburg PA
CBHW061551100726
47898CB00002B/319